FREEDOM FROM DISEASE

FREEDOM
FROM DISEASE

How to control FREE RADICALS, a major cause of aging and disease.

A Scientist Rediscovers
Prevention-Oriented Natural Health Care
MAHARISHI AYUR-VED

by
Hari Sharma, MD

Professor of Pathology and Director,
Cancer Prevention and Natural Products Research,
The Ohio State University, College of Medicine
Columbus, Ohio

VEDA
PUBLISHING

Veda Publishing
Toronto

Published by Veda Publishing, Inc.
Suite 116
65 Front Street West
Toronto, Ontario M5J 1E6
Canada

Manufactured in the United States of America

Canadian Cataloguing in Publication:

Sharma, Hari (Hari M.)
    Freedom from disease: how to control free radicals, a major cause of aging and disease

ISBN 1-895958-00-8

    1. Free radicals (Chemistry)—Physiological effects.
2. Diseases—Causes and theories of causation. 3. Aging—Physiological aspects. 4. Pathology, Molecular. I. Title

RB170.843 1993   616.07´1   C93-090327-7

Cover design and illustration, title page: Bordow Graphics, Inc.
Book design: Robert Oates
Typeface: Janson

Contents

The Book at a Glance

A century ago Louis Pasteur discovered that single-celled microbes cause infectious disease. His discovery triggered the twentieth-century revolution in health.

Now an even more fundamental discovery is producing another health care revolution.

Beyond the single cell, researchers have found *free radicals*—ravenous molecules that damage cells and cripple our health. In the last ten years, these molecular sharks have been identified as a major cause of aging and degenerative disease, and implicated in heart attacks, arthritis, and cancer.

The good news is that such a single cause offers the possibility of a single cure. By controlling free radicals, we should be able to slow the aging process and prevent disease.

Hundreds of scientific studies have shown that free radicals can, in fact, be controlled. Certain drugs and vitamins reduce free radical damage—but uniquely effective control is provided by a prevention-oriented system of natural health care. This much-researched system is *ayurveda*—a comprehensive and integrated approach long preserved in India, and recently revived as Maharishi Ayur-Ved.

Complex herbal food supplements from this traditional health care system have been shown to defuse free radicals 1000 times more effectively than vitamins and a frequently utilized drug. The stress management program that stems from this timeless approach reduces stress more effectively than any other technique so far tested, thus preventing excess free radicals from being created in the first place.

Long-term insurance studies indicate that people who reduce free radical damage through this integrated approach go to the hospital for illness and surgery 80% less than the general population. It appears that our generation can enjoy a quality of health and longevity previously unreported—life with free radicals under control.

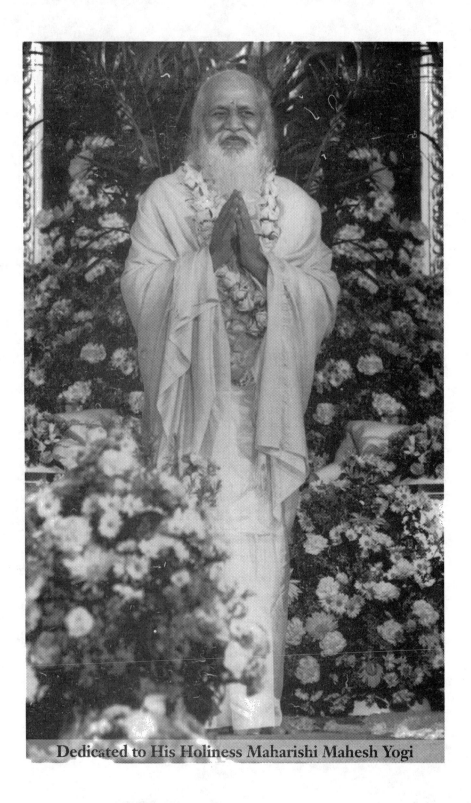

Dedicated to His Holiness Maharishi Mahesh Yogi

Acknowledgments

I must first express my deepest appreciation to Maharishi Mahesh Yogi for his knowledge of consciousness and ayurveda, and the inspiration to write this book. It was he who put me back in touch with my own cultural heritage—the timeless ayurvedic system of prevention-oriented, natural health care long preserved in India.

Next, I would like to thank my family, whose constant patience, love, and support underlie all that I do.

I would also like to thank the many researchers who have worked with me to investigate Maharishi Ayur-Ved, including Chandradhar Dwivedi, Vimal Patel, Kottarappat Dileepan, Rao Panganamala, Howard Newman, Gopi Tejwani, Michael and Susan Dillbeck, Edwards Smith, Charles Alexander, Ralph Stephens, and hundreds of other researchers around the world who are investigating this system of natural health care. I would also like to thank Jeffrey and Rona Abramson and Gerry Bodeker for their constant encouragement, and the Lancaster Foundation, the Abramson Family Foundation, The Bennett Family Foundation, the Bremer Foundation, the Maharishi Ayur-Ved Foundation, and The Ohio State University for their support on many research projects. It is also fitting to honor the many scientists whose research work over the past two decades has established the new free radical paradigm. Many of the leaders in this work are mentioned in the text.

In the preparation of this book, I have received much help for which I am extremely grateful. I must thank Robert and Patricia Oates especially for their editorial assistance at every stage of the project. Ellen Kauffman provided invaluable line editing, and a critical reading by Craig Pearson made a major contribution. Roger Chalmers, Elizabeth Dimock, Kai Drühl, John Fagan, David Orme-Johnson, David Pasco, Keith Wallace, and Ken Walton kindly provided expert attention, and Jacqueline Lee and Greg Poland worked tirelessly on typography. My gratitude for proofing and other timely assistance also goes to Martha Bright, Christy Kleinschnitz, Burton Milward, and Doug Rexford.

Hari Sharma
Columbus, Ohio, USA
May 1, 1993

A Word to the Wise

The scientific discoveries reported in this book can transform human health and health care. Long-term insurance studies show that we can significantly improve our health—and reduce the pressure on our overheated health care system. I am convinced that everyone should be aware of the research reported in this book. This does not mean, however, that people who read this book should try to become medical experts on their own. Nothing in this book is meant to replace the advice of a physician. If you are sick, go to a doctor. In the back of the book, you will find lists of organizations you can contact to find medical doctors who are also familiar with the free radical paradigm and natural prevention. It *is* possible to have the best of both worlds.

INTRODUCTION

The Dual Discovery

This is, first of all, a <u>how-to book</u>: how to <u>avert disease</u>, how to <u>retard aging</u>, how to <u>live a longer and much healthier life</u>.

But this is also a book of scientific discovery. In just the last decade, researchers around the world have defined a new, dual paradigm of human health. The first part of this paradigm concerns *free radicals*—destructive molecular sharks that tear up the cells in our bodies and cause both aging and disease. The second part concerns uniquely effective *control* of free radicals—through a prevention-oriented, consciousness-based system of natural health care.

Most researchers studying free radicals estimate that these deadly molecules help to cause 80% to 90% of the degenerative diseases that afflict the human race. We once thought that cholesterol was a major cause of heart disease, but new research indicates that the real culprits are free radicals. We have long known that arthritis comes from constant inflammation, but free radicals cause such inflammation. It is clear that cancer is caused by gene mutation, but free radicals cause most gene mutation. Where we thought there were many causes, there is often only one.

And to the extent there is a single cause, there can also be a single cure. By controlling free radicals, we should be able to keep ourselves well. Fortunately, long-term insurance studies encourage such optimism. If free radicals help to cause 80% to 90% of degenerative disease, then effective control of free radicals should reduce disease by a like amount. In fact, two insurance studies have indicated that a group of people who control free radicals with the traditional *ayurvedic* health care system of India have reduced their hospitalization for illness and surgery by better than 80% (see Chapter Six for details).

To medical experts not yet conversant with the free radical paradigm, such dramatic health improvements can seem incomprehensible. No other approach to health has ever yielded even a sizeable fraction of such benefits. But a flood of published studies—covered in this book—have redefined the prospects for human health. These studies show that a major cause of disease can be contained—and that much disease then simply disappears. For individuals seeking to stay vital and healthy, for a society being bankrupted by the health care crisis, completely new possibilities have suddenly appeared.

I believe, in fact, that we are in the midst of a medical revolution, the type of transformation that occurs only once every hundred years or so. Hundreds of studies defining this breakthrough have already been published in academic journals—yet the discoveries are not widely understood outside the immediate circle of the researchers themselves. Modern medicine is still trying to cure disease. But the evidence now indicates that a high percentage of disease need never occur at all.

PARADIGM ONE: FREE RADICALS

The first phase of this dual discovery depends on components of our bodies so small and short-lived as to almost evade detection. Molecules are the smallest intact units that structure the human physiology. In this book we will be predominantly concerned with the smallest of the small—infinitesimal two- and three- and four-atom molecules based on oxygen. As we will see in detail, these tiny, oxygen-based molecules—known as free radicals, or oxy radicals—can be devastatingly destructive, wreaking havoc throughout the body. Much of the aging process, as well as the most dire diseases of our time—from arthritis to diabetes, from cardiovascular disease to cancer—stem from the damage caused by these ravaging free radicals.

Free radicals can not only wreak havoc within any given cell. They can also produce serious damage in whole physiological systems. They can cross-link proteins into tangled masses, reducing the flexibility and efficiency of the physical body as a whole. They can help narrow and eventually close arteries leading to the heart, brain, and to every organ and limb—causing slow, cumulative damage or disastrous crises. They can slow down the secretion from the body's glands, starving the body of needed hormones and speeding up the aging process.

Nor can free radicals be entirely avoided. They are an inescapable feature of all oxygen-based life. As a part of the life-giving processes that create energy in every cell, free radicals are created as toxic waste. When the immune system sends special forces to fight infection, free radicals are used as a weapon (and spilled indiscriminately into the environment). If the body takes in pesticides, industrial chemicals, processed foods, cigarette smoke, or alcohol, free radicals are the most common result. And when the mind and body come under stress, free radicals are mass produced.

PARADIGM TWO: CONSCIOUSNESS-BASED HEALTH

The good news is that, if free radicals can't be escaped, they can be controlled. The best news, documented by the long-term studies of insurance statistics, is that controlling free radicals appears to produce a dramatic improvement in the quality of our health.

This second phase of the new health paradigm depends on a level of life even more fundamental than molecules. It actually goes deeper than the atomic and sub-atomic levels as well, and rests on nature's ultimate basis: the unbounded, non-material field that underlies both the physical world and our physical bodies. At this deepest level, twentieth-century physicists have found that solid matter disappears like a desert mirage. The basic building blocks of the universe—protons, electrons, and other sub-atomic particles—dissolve into non-material waves vibrating in an underlying, omnipresent, non-material field. These beautifully complex wave forms, though having no material substance, do exhibit precise orderliness and intelligence. They obey invariant laws of nature that can be described exactly by mathematical formulas cognized within the human awareness. At the immaterial basis of nature, in other words, what remains is a dance of intelligence. The body is based in a field of consciousness (see Chapter Seven).

This underlying dance of intelligence has practical consequences. The research evidence we will review in Part Two shows that free radicals are controlled with unique effectiveness by a natural health care system that takes these realities into account—by a system based on the principles of consciousness. By watering the root of a tree, the entire tree can be affected. By operating from the root layer of the physiology—a layer characterized by intelligence that is deeper than molecules, a layer that is, in fact, the *basis* of atoms and molecules—it is apparently possible to gain control of the molecular sharks.

This knowledge comes from an ancient, prevention-oriented system of natural health care based in the timeless Vedic tradition of India. It is known as *ayurveda*. It has been revived in our time as Maharishi Ayur-Ved and extensively researched through the latest scientific methodologies. The results have challenged our preconceptions.

We can rethink completely what it means to be healthy.

SCIENCE AND BIOGRAPHY

This is a book of science, not biography. But a brief re-counting of my experiences may shed light on the East-West synthesis which, I now believe, promises the greatest possible control of free radical damage. Personally, I did not enter the field of free radical research because I wanted to find the cause of a disease. I entered because I had quite suddenly encountered powerful natural compounds for cure and prevention of disease.

Six years ago, colleagues at several universities joined me in preliminary studies on two natural herbal foods. These were dietary adjuncts prepared according to the ancient recipes of India's traditional system of ayurvedic medicine. The results were extremely encouraging. They indicated that these food supplements fought America's two major killers—by alleviating certain cancer conditions and heart disease risk factors—while they also enlivened specific responses of the immune system, suggesting increased protection against many infectious diseases.

These results were exciting, but puzzling. I have spent a career in Western medicine—allopathic medicine—as both clinical practitioner and research pathologist at The Ohio State University, College of Medicine. There is little precedent in this system of medicine for single substances that produce such profound and wide-ranging effects. The essence of allopathic medicine, in fact, is what has been called the "magic bullet" approach. The doctor waits for symptoms of disease to appear. Then a single drug is sought for each disease, a magic bullet which can be fired at that particular ailment. No such theory of human pathology could explain how one compound could produce so many dramatic health benefits.

That's why I turned to the emerging field of free radical research. Allopathy sees each disease as an isolated phenomenon, requiring a specific treatment. The free radical concept, on the other hand, encourages a fundamental and holistic approach. It allows for a single treatment that can help with a wide range of diseases. It also provides for effective *prevention* of those diseases—a goal not given much consideration in standard allopathy.

As I began to study this single-cause theory, I went through a personal odyssey. I found that the progress of modern medical research had begun to dovetail with understandings and treatments provided by the world's most ancient and multi-faceted system of natural health care. I, who had spent three decades practicing only the Western approach, was suddenly brought face to face with my own cultural heritage—with the traditional ayurvedic health care system long known and practiced in India.

MODERN MEDICINE, ANCIENT MEDICINE

I was born in India, in the city of Aligarh, the province of Uttar Pradesh. At a relatively young age, I knew I wanted a career in medicine. Like many Indians of my generation, I was convinced that the traditional medical knowledge around me was not sufficiently up-to-date and scientific. The Western industrial nations displayed a clear superiority in their material development. It seemed obvious that their scientific, allopathic approach to medicine must also be superior to the traditional, apparently non-scientific medical knowledge available in my homeland. For that reason, I attended a Western-style school of medicine in Lucknow, India, then eventually moved to the United States. My career has been fruitful and fulfilling, and I have never regretted my original decision.

Recent events in my life, however, have caused me to reflect on experiences I had when young. The most important were provided by my father-in-law, who was an ayurvedic physician, or *vaidya* (the first syllable rhymes with *my*: VI-dyuh). He lived in Bareilly, another city in Uttar Pradesh, where I used to visit and watch him practice. He was overwhelmed with patients, surely one index of medical success. I was impressed with how quickly he was able to diagnose underlying problems, using ayurveda's traditional system of pulse diagnosis, and I noted the clinical effectiveness of the herbs he would prescribe for each patient.

I was too much under the spell of the West, however, for his performance to deflect me from my decision. I knew that the Indian government officially supported ayurvedic medicine and research, and that ayurvedic training involved five years of rigorous post-graduate education. I was aware, if only from the experience of my father-in-law, that ayurveda was practiced by intelligent and sophisticated people who enjoyed high levels of success—seemingly without the negative side effects of the allopathic approach. My mind, however, was made up. I left my ayurvedic roots, and I eventually left India for the West.

But life can turn and curl in mysterious ways. Ensconced though I was in mid-career in middle America, my Indian heritage began to catch up with me. This reunion with ayurveda began about a decade ago at Ohio State. First, I learned to practice the Transcendental Meditation technique brought out of India by Maharishi Mahesh Yogi. I began to meditate because I was interested in the evolution of consciousness and spiritual development. But like many researchers, I was attracted to Transcendental Meditation partly by the large body of scientific evidence it had engendered. Repeated studies had shown that the Transcendental Meditation technique reduces stress and anxiety and improves both physical and mental health.

Maharishi himself had been trained as a physicist before turning his attention to meditation, and from the beginning of his teaching in the West he had encouraged scientific investigation of his mental techniques. It was research on his Transcendental Meditation technique, in fact, which first indicated to Western scientists that meditation can have significant positive effects on the human mind and body.

Pleased with the results of my meditation practice, I later found that Maharishi had begun a program of investigation and training in ayurvedic medicine. I was intrigued by this voice from my past. I attended a preliminary training program offered at Maharishi International University, an accredited university located in Fairfield, Iowa. Then I flew to a weekend conference on Maharishi Ayur-Ved held by Western physicians in Boston. Finally, in 1987, I decided to attend an international conference of physicians called by Maharishi and held at his headquarters outside New Delhi, India.

Maharishi had often challenged scientists to research Transcendental Meditation. Now he challenged the physicians at this conference to do research on Maharishi Ayur-Ved. He focused on two herbal formulations known as Maharishi Amrit Kalash (MAK). Derived from recipes handed down by ayurvedic vaidyas through the centuries, MAK is considered a master food supplement. At the conference, in fact, Maharishi said that taking MAK is as important as meditating.

Most of the 150 doctors on the course were physicians in medical practice. I was the only physician there who was also a pathologist, the only one familiar with research protocol. Still, for days I hung back. I wasn't yet convinced that a mixture of Indian herbs was worth the effort involved in major research. But others responded to Maharishi's challenge with research methodologies that I knew to be inadequate. Finally, when I couldn't take it anymore, I spoke up. I was very blunt. "You don't do research like this," I said. I laid out a series of experiments—one, two, three, four—outlining the methodologies necessary to counter skeptical questions and earn academic publication.

"Good," Maharishi said. He smiled. "Now you should do it."

THE BREAKTHROUGH RESEARCH

I felt that I could hardly say no. If Maharishi was willing to submit these ancient formulas to the rigors of modern objective investigation, it didn't seem to me that a responsible investigator should refuse. I had a personal reason as well. A thorough investigation would give me a chance to come to terms with my own heritage. I could apply the experimental skills I had spent a lifetime acquiring to investigate one of the most important promises offered by the traditional medicine of my homeland.

Given the sweeping claims Maharishi had made, I decided that the initial research should look at the effect of MAK on heart disease and cancer, while also testing its impact on the immune system in general. It made sense to find out right away if MAK could make significant inroads on the major health problems. Such an ambitious research program could not be carried out quickly at any one laboratory. For that reason, when I returned to the United States I called around the country to colleagues at other institutions. Researchers at the University of Kansas Medical Center, the South Dakota State University College of Pharmacy, and the Indiana University School of Medicine joined my colleagues at Ohio State in carrying out the research. Within a matter of months those initial experiments had been completed, and all were eventually published in academic journals.

The results, mentioned briefly above, stretched the limits of allopathic common sense. Risk factors for cardiovascular disease were lessened. Certain cancer conditions were alleviated, even reversed. The immune system was strengthened in specific ways—which could improve protection against all infectious illness (see details in Chapter Five). Two herbal foods, composed of natural ingredients and used as a dietary adjunct to the everyday diet, seemed able to offer an unprecedented defense against disease.

When the results of these studies first came in, I did two things. First, to be honest, I added Maharishi Amrit Kalash to my own diet. (So did a number of the other researchers.) Second, I turned my attention to the rapidly growing research literature on free radicals.

The free radical paradigm was the only one I knew that was broad enough to help explain our findings. If a single substance can enliven the immune system, while also affecting the etiology of major illnesses as disparate as heart disease and cancer, only a deeply unified theory of the causes of such disease could help explain our findings. If we had undertaken the MAK research ten years earlier, there might have been no such unified and well-documented understanding available. But the free radical paradigm has now received sufficient empirical verification to make it seem to offer a reasonable explanation.

As we will see in Part Two of this book, there are many ways to fight free radicals effectively. This is the most encouraging aspect of the research. Many substances, including certain drugs, vitamins, bioflavonoids, and other nutrients, have been found to retard the damage caused by free radical attack. But systematic comparative research has indicated that Maharishi Amrit Kalash fights free radicals far more effectively than other substances tested to date.

It is also possible to stop free radicals before they start. In Chapter Two we will see how constant stress and tension cause the body to churn out large numbers of free radicals. Effective stress management can therefore keep free radical levels down. Once again, years of comparative research have shown that the Transcendental Meditation technique—now integrated as a basic approach of Maharishi Ayur-Ved— reduces stress and anxiety more effectively than all other techniques so far tested.

Free radicals are a recent discovery. Their most effective antidotes apparently come from an ancient tradition.

THE BOOK IN BRIEF

To fully appreciate the health possibilities involved in these discoveries, it is necessary to understand the free radical challenge in detail. Why does the body produce within itself molecules that are so self-destructive? How can such tiny molecules cause so much damage? What can we learn about free radical mechanisms that will allow us to nullify their disease-producing effects? The answers to these questions provide a fascinating look into the mechanics of life at the molecular level. They can also generate the motivation to take charge of our own health in simple but effective ways. In the three parts of this book, I have tried to decode the scientific evidence on this topic and put it into simple English:

Part One: The Free Radical Paradigm provides an introductory overview of this new medical model as it has developed in the recent research literature. It explains how free radicals are formed and details specific ways that free radicals hasten the aging process and generate disease.

Part Two: Winning the Battle reviews the research on free radical management. It explains the body's natural defenses against free radicals. It recounts the research on added protection given by pharmaceuticals, vitamins, bioflavonoids, and other nutrients. It also covers in detail the research that changed my career—the research showing that approaches from the ayurvedic tradition, now revived in Maharishi Ayur-Ved, counter free radical damage with unique effectiveness.

Part Three: The Consciousness Paradigm confronts the most important question I have faced in my professional life: Why do food supplements and meditation techniques known for thousands of years fight free radicals more effectively than approaches discovered by modern science? The answer I have come to is this: Consciousness is vital to physical health. The mind is basic to the body. In Part Three, we will explore this topic in detail. We will listen to leading mathematicians and physicists describe their reasons for believing that consciousness is fundamental to the physical world. We will listen to Maharishi Mahesh Yogi as he explains the mechanics by which pure consciousness can self-interact to produce both the world we see and our physical bodies. And we will explore the many approaches of Maharishi Ayur-Ved, a diverse yet integrated system intended to fine-tune both body and mind.

SAVING INDIVIDUALS AND SOCIETIES

Throughout the book, I have included as much of the relevant scientific theory and research as I could, consistent with readability. I believe you can change your life with the facts on free radicals and their antidotes. I also believe that whole societies can profit from this same knowledge. The American government—and all governments—are under attack by free radicals. These are not political radicals, gun-toting and bomb-throwing. They are sub-microscopically small molecules. But when they attack the cells in our bodies, they might just as well be attacking our society with lethal weapons. As they spread disease and dysfunction through the citizens of a nation, they cripple the human resource of that nation—and drain its economic vitality. The health care crisis in America and around the world is caused to a significant degree by the physically crippling depradations of free radicals.

Now we know that we can defend ourselves, individually and as a society. Research has uncovered a new understanding of aging and disease. It appears that we as individuals can dramatically improve our health and longevity—and that we as a society can come to grips with the high cost and indifferent success of our current health care system.

I have written this book to inspire both self-help and social policy.

PART ONE

The Free Radical
Paradigm

CHAPTER ONE

The Health Care Solution

Many physicians, biochemists, and molecular biologists believe that we are witnessing a revolution in medical understanding—a revolution that will wipe out many of our most feared diseases, a revolution that will change forever what it means to grow old. This revolution is based, in the first instance, on a completely new paradigm of aging and disease. It is based on the discovery of organic free radicals.

As with all paradigms, the new free radical explanation of disease and aging amounts to much more than a particular theory. A paradigm is a standpoint, an overall view, a big picture concept that sheds light on the details of any given theory. It is a world view that defines what people are able to think and talk about.

In this case, the new paradigm is based on a deeper penetration into the make-up of the body—a shift of attention to the molecular level of health. It involves the smallest and most fundamental components of our physiology.

This penetration toward the minute began more than a century ago when Louis Pasteur developed the germ theory of disease. His research demonstrated that one-celled microbes, so tiny as to be invisible to the naked eye, can cause large-scale damage in the body. As always with new discoveries, it was years before Pasteur's work was widely accepted. Many doctors could not believe in what they could not see; they did not believe in germs and refused even to wash their hands as they moved from one surgery to another. Pasteur's theory won through, however. Eventually, microbes were battled through medical hygiene and public sanitation, through antibiotics and vaccines, and as a result the twentieth century has enjoyed great gains in health—though Pasteur did not live to see most of the progress his discovery made possible.

Now another such life-enhancing paradigm shift is at hand. As with all true paradigm shifts, the discovery has come from a completely new way of looking at the problem. Pasteur was the first to diagnose disease by focusing down to life's cellular level—using his optical microscope to find uni-cellular organisms that can cause disease. Modern researchers have now focused their attention more deeply. Rather than focusing on organs, or the tissues that make up organs, or even on the cells that make up tissues, the free radical paradigm has moved to the deeper world of molecules and their interactions. Researchers have used today's powerful electron microscopes, electron spin resonance spectrometers, and other modern instruments to probe this fundamental molecular level of life. They have begun to unravel the secrets of biological molecules, so small that billions make up even the smallest cell. And it is this infinitesimal world that harbors free radicals, the molecular terrorists that sabotage our bodies and our health.

The breakthrough is difficult to overestimate. Now researchers have identified a major cause for many of the most serious chronic and degenerative diseases—a major cause for much of what we think of as normal aging and ill health. More significantly, researchers have also identified simple means for slowing and even reversing this damage. With these discoveries serious researchers are suggesting that a life span of 120 years, which now seems the outside human limit enjoyed by only a fabled few, can become routine. The boldest among these experts are even suggesting that the maximum life span could be increased to 150 years and beyond. And those interested in this field are not just speaking of being *old* longer. They are speaking of being *young* longer—of enjoying the appearance, physical energy, and mental clarity of youth well into what is now called old age.

THE NEED OF OUR TIME

For those of us who have devoted our lives to modern medical science, this fundamental new approach to health has come at a propitious moment. As the mass media never let us forget, the modern health care system has slipped into a deepening crisis. As this book goes to press, Americans are spending more than $800 billion a year on health care, nearly three times what they spend on national defense, more than 14% of the nation's gross national product. Management experts predict that within a decade, health care costs will cancel all corporate profits and bring the capitalist economy to a halt.

Moreover, a growing consensus in society indicates that the basic premises of modern health care may need revising. The allopathic approach waits for symptoms of disease to arise, then brings to bear a vast armory of machinery, drugs, surgical procedures, and hospital equipment to fight the symptoms and/or the causes as they appear. As medical research progresses, more and more costly machinery, surgical procedures, and drug interventions proliferate. No one wants to deny any ill patient the latest and most expensive treatments available— and the costs have escalated out of control.

The most tragic aspect of the modern approach, however, to the great sorrow of the dedicated medical practitioners who wish to bring good health to their patients, is that the allopathic system is itself a major cause of ill health and disease. It is well known, for example, that most surgical procedures weaken patients' resistance and predispose to further illness, even when the surgery itself is successful. Worse, the surgery itself can go awry, causing major damage. In addition, diagnostic procedures such as cardiac catheterization and hemodialysis are increasingly invasive and dangerous. Finally, the side effects of drugs are notoriously damaging, especially if many drugs are prescribed simultaneously.

The dangers of the allopathic approach were rigorously shown in a landmark research study published a decade ago. This study sobered medical specialists more than anything that had appeared previously because it was conducted by physicians at a large university hospital and published by the premier medical journal, the *New England Journal of Medicine*. The study tracked every patient admitted to the general medical service of that hospital over a five-month period—815 patients in all—and counted the total number of iatrogenic ("physician-induced") diseases contracted by those patients during their hospital stay. The study was conservatively done. In the words of the authors, "If there was even slight reason to believe that an event reflected the natural progression of a disease, it was not included [as iatrogenic]."

Despite this conservative approach, the results were disheartening. More than one-third of all patients, 36%, were listed as contracting at least one iatrogenic disease while in the hospital. The majority of these diseases were caused by drugs and drug interactions (a study twenty years earlier had tracked only iatrogenic illnesses caused by drugs, and the percentages of drug-induced disease in the two studies were nearly identical). Nearly 10% of the patients contracted a serious iatrogenic disease, defined as a disease that was life-threatening or that created a major disability. Two per cent of the patients, one in 50 hospital admissions in this study, died in situations caused or complicated by iatrogenic disease.[1]

BEYOND MEDICINE TO PREVENTION

As I can tell you personally, statistics like these are deeply depressing to those in the medical profession. Practicing physicians spend long years in medical school, work to stay abreast of the latest research and procedures, apply their knowledge with all the focus and concern they can muster— then watch as their efforts produce disease in a discouragingly high percentage of those who come for their care. Those who work in the laboratories to come up with better cures have also felt frustrated as their labors have not produced more uniformly encouraging results. With far too many diseases, as critics have bitterly said, "The physician is the pathogen."

There could be a simple solution to all of this, if only it were possible: Ideally we would be able to prevent illness before it begins. Once patients fall ill, physicians find it difficult to resist playing Russian roulette with the modern medical approaches—hoping each time that the cure will appear without the complications. But if people could simply stay healthy, both the dangers and the costs of modern health care would be significantly reduced.

Unfortunately, keeping people healthy has appeared a daunting task. Exercise and diet control have been proven effective, but it is hard to get people to change their habits. Avoiding carcinogens in the environment would surely be a good idea, but there is no easy way to do this. Being calm and happy correlates with health and long life, but how do you alter a person's personality? Prevention is the health care goal of the Nineties, but where can you find an effective yet easy approach to prevention?

Now the discovery of free radicals in every living cell has led to a practical and powerful new approach to prevention. It's a new paradigm, well established experimentally, but just barely finding its way into doctors' offices and the popular press. The health-maintaining effects appear extremely powerful, yet the procedures are easy.

To live a long life in good health, you must control the free radicals unleashed in your body.

INFECTION AND DEGENERATION

Pasteur's discovery of microbes produced a remarkable improvement in human health. Infectious diseases such as tuberculosis and pneumonia nearly disappeared in developed nations. Largely as a result, the average life span in the United States increased from 49 at the turn of the century to 76 today. But this great progress did not produce perfectly healthy human beings. Instead, with the reduction of infectious diseases, new diseases became more prominent—diseases that appeared to come from within. These are the chronic and degenerative diseases such as heart disease, cancer, kidney failure, diabetes, arthritis, and the host of other maladies that now afflict people in the industrialized nations. These chronic and degenerative diseases are no less crippling and lethal than infectious diseases. But their causes have seemed more complex and elusive, and their prevention more difficult.

Also exposed to view by the decline of infectious diseases was the mysterious process of aging. As more and more people lived longer and longer, the intrinsic damage done by "natural aging" was more widely studied. In this case, as well, the causes seemed difficult to define. The DNA molecule at the core of every cell is so effective at repairing and replacing its components that it appears essentially immortal—being passed for millennia from one generation to the next. In addition, any individual cell in the human body is well equipped with systems to repair and replace its constituent parts in a seemingly endless process. In the words of Elliott Crooke, a biochemist at Georgetown University, "Protein turnover and replacement [in the cell] is an effective and faithful system that is designed to last forever."[2]

In the face of these apparently ageless mechanisms, the body is still seen to age in obvious ways. The skin wrinkles.

The hair whitens. Muscles waste and ligaments stiffen. Chronic and degenerative diseases set in and progressively worsen. Eventually, even in the best of cases, the body's mechanisms cease to function in fundamental ways and it "dies of natural causes."

But what causes this progressive spread of dysfunction? Until recently, no one had a well-documented answer. In the absence of more logical explanations, researchers began to postulate ideas seemingly better suited to science fiction. They envisioned "suicide genes" in the DNA or "suicide hormones" produced in the neuroendocrine system. They imagined the body a ticking time bomb set to destroy itself. But up to now, such self-destructive genes or hormones have not been located.

THE OXYGEN PARADOX

Over the past decade, the free radical paradigm has helped solve this mystery of illness and aging. And the basic realization underlying the free radical paradigm is that oxygen, the atmospheric source of life, is also a source of degeneration, disease and, ultimately, death.

We live surrounded by and suffused with oxygen. We take it completely for granted, walk through it thoughtlessly, breathe it in, sometimes greedily. Now, as if we suddenly discovered that water kills fish, we have discovered that oxygen kills cells, tissues, and, eventually, the entire body.

The two-edged nature of oxygen is known as the *oxygen paradox*. On the one hand, oxygen bestows life-giving energy. Without oxygen a living cell can still extract energy from glucose molecules through anaerobic metabolism (anaerobic means "without air," or, more precisely, "not in the presence of oxygen"). With oxygen, however, the body can extract sixteen times as much energy from the same number of glucose molecules. Given the energy demands on the human system, the difference is life and death. Neurons in the brain are especially energy sensitive, and even minutes of oxygen starvation lead to rapid neuron death.

On the other hand, as a moment's reflection reveals, oxygen is extremely corrosive. A fine new automobile, left to the mercies of oxygen, will eventually rust down to a pile of dust. Oxygen spoils food, turns butter rancid, even eats the granite in our grandest mountains. Given the slightest opportunity, moreover, oxygen will burn to cinders anything flammable.

The essential insight of the new free radical paradigm is that oxygen, if given the chance, destroys the molecular components of the body just as surely as it rusts metal and burns buildings. At its most destructive, oxygen combines with hydrogen into various unstable and highly reactive free radical molecules, as well as other *reactive oxygen species* (ROS). In these virulent forms, oxygen will systematically destroy a cell's DNA, enzymes, proteins, and membranes—unless the body's defenses keep the attack in check.

This is the dark side of oxygen. Seen from the most extreme point of view, in fact, oxygen is a poison gas. Anyone who breathes pure oxygen for 48 hours will die, a victim of oxygen's damage to the tissues of the lung. Living in the earth's atmosphere, we continue to survive only because inert nitrogen dilutes oxygen down to 20% of the air we breathe— and the body has developed coping mechanisms to counter oxygen's destructive effects at levels this low.

Our use of oxygen is thus a Faustian bargain—a life-giving boon with a lethal curse attached. Oxygen powers the chemical reactions that provide energy for motion, sensation, and thought—for all that makes possible animal and human life on this planet. But the oxygen that saturates our cells is also a constant threat to our survival. It mounts a relentless attack that eventually wears down our defenses and destroys our biological machinery. The body gets old because, in large part, oxygen wastes it away. The body suffers from a heart attack, or a stroke, or an outbreak of cancer because, in large part, oxygen has done its damage. Oxygen gives life, and oxygen takes it away.

A DESTRUCTIVE HUNGER

Why is oxygen, so necessary to life, also so destructive? The driving force in both cases, as we will see in Chapter Two, must be explained in atomic and sub-atomic terms. The central idea can be stated simply: Oxygen has an elemental hunger for electrons.

Electrons are the negatively charged particles that swirl rapidly around every atom's nucleus. When two or more atoms link up as a molecule, some of the now common electrons circumnavigate the entire molecule. Certain atoms and molecules have their electrons nicely balanced and demonstrate great stability in their structure. They are not interested in reacting with other atoms or molecules. However, if electrons are configured in an uneven or unbalanced way, the atoms or molecules are unstable. They want to abduct nearby electrons to resolve their own internal imbalances.

Even by itself, oxygen is relatively unstable and eager to confiscate electrons from other atoms or molecules. Combined variously with hydrogen, oxygen produces several small molecules even more voracious in their electron appetite. These are dangerous free radical molecules, also known as *oxy radicals*.

All free radicals are one electron short. Their drive to even up this imbalance sends them in frenzied attacks against their molecular neighbors. This is especially true of the small, mobile, and highly reactive oxy radicals. Other atomic and molecular varieties of oxygen are known as reactive oxygen species (ROS). These are not technically free radicals, but they are nonetheless unstable and highly reactive with the molecules around them.

These oxy radicals and ROS can become terrorists in our physical bodies. They can attack DNA, leading to dysfunction, mutation, and cancer. They can attack enzymes and proteins, disrupting normal cell activities. They can attack cell membranes, producing a chain reaction of destruction; such membrane damage in the cells that line our blood vessels can lead to hardening and thickening of the arteries and eventually to heart attacks and strokes. Free radical attacks on the protein in collagen can cause cross-linking of protein molecules and a resulting stiffness in the body. Excess free radical activity in the skin, caused by radiation from the sun, can reduce skin suppleness and increase wrinkling.

The list of diseases now linked to oxy radicals and ROS is long and disturbing:

•Cancer

•Arteriosclerosis, atherosclerosis

•Heart disease

•Strokes

•Emphysema

•Maturity onset diabetes (the most common diabetes)

•Rheumatoid arthritis

•Ulcers

•Cataracts

•Crohn's disease

•Behcet's disease

•Reynaud's disease

•Senility

As already indicated, the oxygen onslaught also helps to cause many of the less serious but still bedeviling symptoms of aging: wrinkled and unresilient skin, gray hair and balding, and bodily stiffness. Oxy radicals and ROS have even been linked to such minor but embarrassing conditions as dandruff and hangovers. One of the most experienced researchers in the field, Japanese biochemist Yukie Niwa, estimates that at least 85% of chronic and degenerative diseases are the result of oxidative damage.[3]

An increasing flood of research is demonstrating that *oxidative stress*—the constant attack by oxy radicals and reactive oxygen species—is important in both the initiation and promotion stages of many major diseases. They help cause the disease in the first place, then add impetus to its spread in the body. With heart disease, as we will see, oxidative stress can cause major damage even after treatment has been applied.

THE POSITIVE SIDE

Despite the lengthy list of problems they cause, free radicals are not all bad. They have vital roles to play in a healthy human body. In the first place, certain types of free radicals are integral to nearly every chemical reaction that occurs in the body. The body constantly needs to create complex new molecules from pieces of old ones. Every time the body's enzymes help an organic molecule to be broken apart and recombined, the intermediary molecular pieces can lose one or more electrons. Frequently this makes them free radicals.

However, these molecular pieces are typically large, composed of thousands and even tens of thousands of atoms. Their large size renders them relatively immobile and unreactive. In addition, the enzymes in charge of the reaction usually keep a solid grip on these molecular fragments until they see them safely attached to their destined partner. Once the new combination is formed, all electron hungers have been satisfied and the danger of free radical damage has passed.

Second, the body actually attempts to harness the destructive power of the most dangerous free radicals—the small and highly reactive oxy radicals and reactive oxygen species—for use in the immune system and inflammatory reactions. Certain cells in these systems first engulf invading bacteria or viruses. Then they take up oxygen molecules from the bloodstream, create a flood of oxy radicals and ROS, and bombard the invader with this toxic shower.

To an impressive degree, this aggressive use of toxic oxygen species succeeds in protecting the body against dangerous invaders. Unfortunately, however, the process can easily get out of control, as we will see in Chapter Three.

THE CAUSES OF FREE RADICALS

Production of free radicals in the body is continuous and inescapable. We will discuss the mechanisms in detail in the next chapter, but the basic categories can be listed briefly:

Energy production: The energy-producing process in every cell generates oxy radicals and ROS as toxic waste—continuously and in abundance. Oxygen is used to burn glucose molecules that act as the body's fuel. In this energy-freeing operation, oxy radicals are thrown off as destructive by-products. Given the insatiable electron hunger of oxygen, there is no way to have it suffusing the body's energy-producing processes without the constant creation of oxy radicals and ROS.

Immune system: As we have just seen, immune system cells create oxy radicals and ROS deliberately, as weapons.

Pollution and other external substances: In modern life, we are constantly exposed to external substances which generate free radicals in the body. Once ingested, for example, many farm chemicals, including fertilizers and pesticides, produce free radicals as by-products. The same is true for many prescription drugs; the harmful side effects of many drugs are caused by the free radicals they generate. Processed foods frequently contain high levels of lipid peroxides, which produce free radicals that damage the cardiovascular system. Cigarette smoke generates high free radical concentrations; the lung damage associated with smoking is largely caused by free radicals. The same is true of environmental pollution. Alcohol is also a particularly virulent free radical generator. In addition, all types of electromagnetic radiation can cause free radicals—including, unfortunately, sunlight. When sunlight hits the skin, it generates free radicals which then age the skin with roughness and wrinkles. If the exposure is severe enough, skin cancer can result.

Stress: The fast pace of modern life is also a recipe for free radicals. The constant pressure and time-shortage experienced by most people in industrialized countries causes them to experience high levels of stress. And stress in the body creates free radicals in abundance. It races the body's energy-creating apparatus, increasing the number of free radicals created as toxic waste. Moreover, the hormones which cause the stress reaction in the body come to a bad end; they themselves degenerate into particularly destructive free radicals. Researchers now know why stress creates disease. A stressful life mass produces free radicals.

FREE RADICAL DEFENSES

Given the many sources of free radicals, all aerobic forms of life maintain elaborate anti-free radical defense systems (also known as *anti-oxidant* systems).

Enzymes: Every cell in the body creates its own "bomb squad"—anti-oxidant enzymes (complex, machine-like proteins) whose particular job it is to defuse oxy radicals and ROS. One of the most destructive free radicals, for example, is superoxide. The most thoroughly-studied defense enzyme, known as superoxide dismutase, takes hold of superoxide molecules and changes them to a much less reactive form.

Nutrients: As the second tier of defense, the body makes use of many standard vitamins and other nutrients, including vitamins C and E, beta-carotene, bioflavonoids, and many others, to quench the oxy radicals' destructive thirst for electrons. Many free radical researchers feel that to fight free radicals effectively the general levels of all these free radical-fighting nutrients need to be much higher than nutritional experts previously thought.

Self-repair: In addition to using enzymes and nutrients for direct attacks on oxy radicals, the body also has a rapid and thorough system to repair and/or replace damaged building blocks of the cell. For example, the system for repairing damage to the DNA and other nucleic acids is particularly elaborate and efficient. The process involves separate specific enzymes which first locate damaged areas, then snip out ruined bits, replace them with the correct sequence of molecules, and seal up the strand once again. Every aspect of the cell is given similar attention. Most protein constituents in the cell, for example, are completely replaced every few days. Scavenger enzymes break used and damaged proteins into their component parts for reuse by the cell.

These elaborate biochemical responses to the free radical challenge suggest that it is not necessary to reduce the body's excess free radicals to zero. *The body need only strike a proper balance between the number of free radicals generated and the defense and repair mechanisms available.* The goal is to keep oxidative stress below the level at which normal repair and replacement can maintain 100% cell efficacy. Oxy radicals might slip through the enzyme and nutrient defenses to attack the DNA, for instance. But, ideally, these attacks would be few enough that the DNA repair mechanisms could fix the damage and maintain the genetic code intact.

As we will see in Chapter Six, such a healthful internal balance is possible—with dramatic effects on health and health care costs.

THE MOST FUNDAMENTAL THEORY

It's an exciting time in medical history. In addition to the free radical breakthrough, other approaches to slowing aging are also being tried. Two of these have been widely publicized.

The first approach is hormone therapy. At Veterans Administration Hospitals in Milwaukee and Chicago, twenty-seven elderly volunteers have tried weekly injections of genetically engineered growth hormone. Preliminary results indicate an increase of physical strength and energy.

The second approach uses calorie restriction. In many scientific laboratories, the life span of animals has been extended, sometimes nearly doubled, by reducing their daily intake of food drastically. The National Institutes of Health are now putting $30 million into a long-term test with humans to see the result of significant calorie restriction in the daily diet.

In my view, however, developing strategies for free radical management offers the most hope—with the least chance for negative side effects—while also providing the chance to enjoy the benefits of these other approaches as well. In the first place, given medical history, it seems unlikely that we can use laboratory-developed hormones for frequent injection without the creation of long-term difficulties. The trials with growth hormone so far have resulted in at least one troubling side effect: inflammation of joints. It also seems to me that extra years bought as the result of near-starvation might seem more punishment than blessing.

Most significantly, however, successful free radical management may make both these approaches unnecessary. Studies by biochemist Richard Cutler of the National Institute on Aging suggest that free radical damage slows down hormone secretion in the major glands. As internal hormone production slows down, injection of hormones may have a noticeable effect. We could obviate the need for hormone injections, however, if we could stave off free radical attack and keep our glands at maximum efficiency. Already, research on Maharishi Ayur-Ved has shown that it helps maintain high levels of dehydroepiandrosterone sulfate (DHEA-S), the most widely circulated hormone in the body (see Chapter Six).[4]

As for caloric restriction, the most likely reason that metabolizing less food increases life span is the correlation between metabolism and free radical production. If you burn less food, you create fewer oxy radicals. The same result, however, could be theoretically achieved without the need to court starvation—by eating a healthy diet and then managing the resultant free radicals more successfully. As we will see, humans as a species have already increased their peak caloric intake by four times over many other mammals by increasing their capability for neutralizing free radicals. There seems no reason why life span can't be further increased by increasing anti-oxidant levels within the body.

This is not to say that the free radical challenge is easily met. The difficulty would not be so great if the only free radical sources were the immune system and the energy-creating process in every cell. Unfortunately, this is not the case. The body may be holding its own against the inevitable free radicals produced by natural physiological processes—but new onslaughts caused by environmental pollution and stressful living can tip the balance. Since the modern industrial environment is so heavily polluted, there seems no short-term escape from this externally caused onslaught. Since the pace of modern life seems only to speed up, there also seems to be no way to avoid constant pressure and tension. This only makes it seem more likely that the body needs help in its constant struggle against oxidative stress. We must put ourselves in the position to help supplement the body's natural defenses. The pioneers in free radical research have gone a long way toward making that possible.

A HISTORY OF PROMISE

When future medical history books are written, one man will be recognized as the first free radical pioneer. He is Dr.

Denham Harman, now nearing 80 years of age, Professor Emeritus of Medicine and Biochemistry at the University of Nebraska. As long ago as 1954, Dr. Harman published a paper implicating free radicals as a major cause of aging and disease. But as with Pasteur and many other pioneers, his ideas went unheeded for many years. Most medical specialists and gerontologists had not yet shifted their attention down to the molecular level, and to them Harman's argument sounded far-fetched.

Eventually, however, Harman's ideas were picked up—not by medical researchers but by biochemists and molecular biologists. Two of the key investigators were Joseph McCord and Irwin Fridovich. First, in 1969, McCord and Fridovich published research showing that living cells contain the free radical-fighting enzyme superoxide dismutase (SOD).[5] Until then, most researchers thought that free radicals did not exist in human and animal cells. But if SOD was in the cell, then surely superoxide must be there as well.

A decade later, McCord and Fridovich published research that broke the field wide open. They demonstrated for the first time that free radicals can be responsible for major damage to cells and whole physiological systems. Their studies demonstrated the reality of *reperfusion injury* to the heart, severe coronary damage that happens after a heart attack has been treated. When doctors use new drugs such as streptokinase to dissolve the blood clot that is preventing blood from reaching the heart muscle, the sudden flood of oxygen returning to the cells causes an explosion of oxy radicals and ROS. Lulled by the previous absence of oxygen, the cells aren't ready for the sudden attack. Serious damage is done in seconds. When McCord and Fridovich demonstrated the reality of such reperfusion injury in animals, the free radical theory moved to the forefront in laboratories around the country.[6]

Oxy radicals and ROS typically live only millionths of a second before biting into another molecule. It is hard to catch them in the act. One of the first to do so was Dr. Donald Malins of the Pacific Northwest Research Foundation in Seattle. He found the first direct evidence that free radicals cause cancer. One in nine American women contract breast cancer, and one in four who contract it is killed by it. Dr. Malins looked at the DNA in human breast cancer cells. There, attached to the DNA, he found spent hydroxy radical molecules, the most ravenous type of oxy radical. Here was the first smoking gun—clear evidence that the cancerous mutation of the DNA had been caused by free radical attack.[7]

Over the course of the 1980s, intriguing evidence continued to pile up. Researchers found a bacteria that could exist in the seemingly lethal environment created by radioactive waste water. Such high levels of radioactivity cause cascades of free radicals in a living cell, one of the mechanisms by which radioactivity kills most forms of life. But the strangely durable bacteria, named *Micrococcus radiodurans*, was found to have three times as much SOD as other microbes, and fifty times as much catalase, another free radical-fighting enzyme. *Micrococcus radiodurans* was apparently surviving by mopping up free radicals as fast as they were generated.[8]

Another encouraging finding came from the laboratories of Dr. John Carney at the University of Kentucky in Lexington. Dr. Carney and his colleagues compared the ability of young and old gerbils to learn a complex maze. At first, the elderly gerbils made 2.5 times more mistakes than the young ones. The elderly gerbils were also found to have lower levels of neurotransmitters—the biochemicals that allow brain cells to communicate—and their neurons were found to have high concentrations of crippled proteins damaged by free radicals. The elderly gerbils were then given an industrial anti-oxidant (oxy radical quencher), known as *N-tert-butyl-alpha-phenyl-nitrone* (PBN). The results were startling. The neurotransmitter levels in the mature gerbils rose markedly, the level of damaged proteins returned to normal and, most significantly, the elderly gerbils began to run the maze almost as well as the youngsters. Slowing the damage done by free radicals apparently allowed brain cells to return to near-optimal functioning. Here was evidence that symptoms of aging and senility could actually be reversed.[9]

FREE RADICAL MANAGEMENT

Much of the research on free radicals now focuses not on what they do, but on how to manage them. Though some researchers want to examine in finer detail the mechanisms by which free radicals cause aging and disease (see Chapter Three for more details), many others feel that we don't really need more information about the problem. What we need is a solution. It seems clear that the human free radical-quenching system may need supplementation—help from outside—to deal with the constant pressure of oxidative stress. Thus, many of the recent research studies focus on ways to add strength to the body's own free radical defenses. There are three broad areas to this research.

Pharmaceutical anti-oxidants: First, not surprisingly, much research is being done on anti-free radical drugs. Research done by the major pharmaceutical companies in their own labs, or university research funded by them, aims at the discovery of pharmaceutical agents that can quench free radicals without otherwise damaging the body. The studies have used industrial anti-oxidants such as PBN, as well as probucol and other such chemicals. One aim has been to find an anti-oxidant drug that can be administered immediately before anti-clotting agents, to prevent reperfusion injury to the heart caused by free radicals.

Enhancing enzymes: Another line of chemical research is attempting to either mimic or enhance the natural anti-oxidant activity of the body's own enzymes. SOD, for example, is a spectacularly effective anti-oxidant enzyme. But SOD can't be absorbed in the body when taken by mouth; the stomach's digestive enzymes break it down. It is also difficult to inject SOD effectively because it has only a brief half-life in the bloodstream. In less than five minutes, 50% of it is gone, broken down by natural bodily processes. Within an hour, only 0.1% of the original concentration still exists. Recently, however, Japanese researcher Tatsuya Oda found a way around this half-life problem. He has succeeded in attaching SOD to artificial polymer molecules. Riding on the polymers, SOD persists in the bloodstream for at least five hours. Dr. Oda has used this polymerized SOD successfully in rats to prevent the lethal free radical effects produced by influenza.[10]

Nutrient anti-oxidants: Despite some initial successes in such drug research, however, many of the leading researchers in the field are focusing on more natural approaches. There are two reasons for this. First, pharmaceuticals have a long history of producing unforeseen and often calamitous side effects. Who knows, for example, the long-term effects of artificially maintaining high levels of SOD in the blood? The body must have some reason for rapidly clearing this useful enzyme—but no one knows yet what it is. Too often, the answers to such questions appear 20 years later in seriously debilitating side effects among people who have used the drug.

Second, the interest in natural anti-oxidants also stems simply from the fact that the body uses so many of them itself. Vitamins C and E, the B vitamin complex, bioflavonoids, and other such relatively small-molecule nutrients have all been shown to play major roles in the body's anti-oxidant defenses. The advantages of these nutrients are easy to enumerate. All of them can be taken by mouth. All of them are familiar to every cell in the body. Receptors located on cell membranes recognize them, and the body can make use of most of them in large doses with virtually no side effects. The only questions seem to be which nutrients to take, in what combination, and in what doses?

These questions are now mainstream science, as illustrated by a recent $17 million research grant from the National Institutes of Health. The grant funds a five-year study of 40,000 women to test the long-term effects of vitamin E and beta-carotene on heart disease and cancer.

ARTIFICIAL OR NATURAL NUTRIENTS?

There is still a split among researchers interested in this nutrient approach. One group advocates artificial vitamins and another prefers the same nutrients in a naturally occurring form. Each has logic on its side. Those who experiment with and recommend artificial vitamins point out that ascorbic acid (vitamin C), for instance, is always molecularly identical—whether it is taken from an orange or synthesized in a laboratory. If the body is comfortable with such a molecule, what difference does it make how the molecule originated? Research on artificial vitamins has clearly shown that they can have anti-oxidant effects in the body.

Advocates of naturally produced nutrients point out, however, that the body is not a one-note instrument. Instead, it is a symphony of complex and interrelated harmonies—the mysteries of which researchers have barely begun to unravel. In an orange, for example, ascorbic acid is accompanied by a complex of up to 100 other nutrients known as bioflavonoids. Theoretically, any or all of these could help ascorbic acid be assimilated into the bloodstream, or be recognized and taken into the cell, or they could themselves be useful co-workers (co-factors) in the anti-oxidant process. In fact, many of these bioflavonoids have already been shown to have anti-oxidant properties themselves (see Chapter Four). It could take decades to gain even a general notion of what all these properties and interactions might be. Meanwhile, we know that the human body is set up to use naturally occurring ascorbic acid in concert with its bioflavonoid cohorts. Why not take the chance on increased benefits?

There is no shortage of these naturally occurring free radical scavengers. Plants are a rich source of such anti-oxidants. Because plants create oxygen as a by-product of harnessing the sun's energy through photosynthesis, they have had to develop powerful anti-oxidant defenses to combat the lethal combination of sunlight and oxygen. Sunlight plus oxygen is a recipe for free radicals. The anti-oxidant substances used by plants to control these free radicals work equally well in the human body. To researchers who emphasize points such as these, natural nutrients recommend themselves as both plentiful and safe—and their rich biodiversity offers the possibility of many as yet undiscovered synergistic benefits.

Research conducted on Maharishi Amrit Kalash (MAK-4 and MAK-5), the two herbal food supplements mentioned in the Introduction, has strongly supported the natural view. At Ohio State we compared the free radical-fighting ability of MAK to known anti-oxidant substances. Compared weight-to-weight with vitamins C and E, and a frequently researched anti-oxidant drug (probucol), both MAK-4 and MAK-5 were far more effective—MAK-4 more than a thousand times (see Chapter Five for details).

ONE CAUSE, ONE CURE

All aspects of the free radical paradigm are now well understood. It is a story that hinges on nature's subtle mechanics. The agglomeration of atoms into molecules is based on the nature and flow of the electrons that whirl about them. The unbalanced hunger and consequent destruction caused by oxy radicals and ROS has everything to do with the subtle and sometimes paradoxical qualities displayed by the most thoroughly studied of all sub-atomic particles, the electron. These deepest secrets of nature's sub-atomic functioning, once the province of physicists alone, now help explain why the flu causes aches and pains, why hair turns gray, and why hearts grow weak. Good health, we now find, depends on the sub-atomic world. Physicians can now learn from physicists.

This radically new view of health science may seem at first intimidatingly complex. Actually, it has resulted in a great simplification. When we think of the thousands of different diseases humanity is heir to, it can seem a hopeless task to study and solve them all. If we imagine a single and unique cause for each single disease, the chase for cures can seem unending. But if we shift our focus to a deeper level of nature's functioning, and find one overall mechanism that helps cause and exacerbate the large majority of such diseases, then this can give great hope.

It is true that the free radical evidence compiled in the laboratories is just now beginning to seep out into hospitals and doctor's offices. This is no surprise. There is ordinarily a ten- to thirty-year gap between major medical discoveries and their practical use by medical professionals. As a pathologist, I have witnessed this gap between basic science and clinical practice throughout my career. Pathologists are medical doctors, some of whom focus primarily on research into causes and cures. Clinical practitioners, on the other hand, focus primarily on each patient who comes through the door. There is a gap between the two. It can take time to get important discoveries out of the lab and into the clinics.

This is especially true if the discovery is revolutionary. In this case, the dramatically new free radical paradigm forces physicians to think on a deeper level of the physiology than their training has prepared them for. It also requires them to shift their attention from, primarily, diagnosis and cure to, primarily, prevention. The change is great and it is not surprising that it hasn't been adopted everywhere immediately.

Fortunately, however, this is one revolution where individuals can do much for themselves. It is true that the entire society will gain the maximum benefit only when free radical management becomes a top priority for physicians everywhere. But we can all take simple steps right now to reduce the damage that is otherwise inevitable. To a degree heretofore unprecedented, good health is in our own hands.

In Part Two, we will discuss the research on free radical management—and the spectacular improvements it brings to health (and health care costs). It is an encouraging prospect. Before we explore what could be the solution, however, it makes sense to more thoroughly understand the problem. What are free radicals? How are they created? How do they cause damage? The answers lie at the sub-microscopic level of life, where electrons, atoms, and molecules dance in a paradoxical realm.

Notes

1. Steel K, et al, *New Eng J Med* 304(1981): 638-42

2. Elliot Crooke, Asst. Prof. of Biochemistry at Georgetown University, personal communication (December, 1992)

3. NiwaY, Hanssen M, *Protection for Life: How to Boost your Body's Defences Against Free Radicals and the Ageing Effects of Pollution and Modern Lifestyles* (Thorsons Publishers, Ltd., Wellingborough, 1989), p. 9

4. Glaser JL, et al, *J Behav Med* 15(1992): 327-41

5. Hooper C, *J NIH Res* 1(1989): 101-6

6. McCord JM, Roy RS, *Can J Physiol Pharmacol* 60(1982): 1346-52

7. Malins DC, Haimanot R, *Cancer Res* 51(1991): 5430-2

8. Driedger AA, et al, *Radiat Research* 44(1970): 835-45

9. Carney JM, et al, *Proc Nat'l Acad Sci USA* 88(1991): 3633-6

10. Oda T, et al, *Science* 244(1989): 974-6

CHAPTER TWO

How Free Radicals Are Created

In the next two chapters, we will take a closer look at free radicals—how they are created and what damage they do. Like any excursion into the mechanics of life, this topic has intrinsic interest. We live our lives among large-scale objects, among chairs and tables, television sets and automobiles. It is fascinating to contemplate the infinitesimal world at the basis of it all—the molecular world where everything depends on the fate of single electrons.[1]

There is, moreover, another reason to pay attention. Free radicals, their genesis, and their destructive ways can teach us things that make a difference. Research evidence indicates that we can live longer, healthier, happier lives by taking simple steps to stop free radical damage. Like Ebenezer Scrooge facing the spirits of Christmas, if we face the reality of free radicals, we can gain motivation to change our ways.

THE FREE RADICAL WORLD

Free radicals live in a different world. It is a world unimaginably minute, where molecules and occasional free atoms are all that exist. To give some idea of scale, one-twelfth of a cup of water contains 6×10^{23} molecules. That's 600,000,000,000,000,000,000,000—or sixty billion trillion—molecules. To equal the number of molecules in this sip of water, you must multiply the human population on earth (5.5 billion) by a little more than ten trillion.

At body temperature, this populous molecular environment displays incessant, frenetic activity. Heat is actually molecules in motion. The molecules in warm air rising from a heater are bouncing off each other more frantically than molecules in cold air—giving extra stimulation to nerve cells in the body, which registers as the sensation of heat. Within a living cell, the rate of activity is so rapid as to challenge comprehension. Imagine an aerial view of the intense automobile and pedestrian traffic in New York City—speeded up millions of times. That's what life is like inside every cell of your body.

All this activity has a purpose. The faster the molecules collide, the more quickly they react with each other—joining together or splitting apart. Thus, heat (molecular motion) increases the speed of molecular reactions. At 98.6° Fahrenheit, molecules jostle one another at the proper intensity to stimulate the biochemical reactions necessary for human life.

THE CELL: A BIOLOGICAL CITY-STATE

The cell is the smallest self-sufficient unit of life. It can carry out all the processes necessary to life—including energy creation, self-maintenance, and reproduction. In a sense, the cell is halfway between molecules and humanity. Cells are composed of molecules. We are composed of cells.

To speak metaphorically, each cell is a walled city-state. It has a governmental building (the nucleus) housing the governing body (*deoxyribonucleic acid*, or DNA). It has power houses (mitochondria), manufacturing centers (Golgi apparatus and ribosomes), an infrastructure (internal membranes, cytoskeleton, and cytosol), and trash disposal (lysosomes). All this is enclosed within the city wall—a semi-permeable membrane. The cell also has elaborate communications systems and a sophisticated import-export mechanism, both of which function within and across the cell membrane.

Like any city-state, the cell can be challenged by destructive agents within. In this case the subversive forces are free radicals. To stop free radical terrorism, every cell has alert anti-free radical forces on constant patrol. The miraculously complex systems within the cell are extremely delicate. They must be protected through the tireless vigilance of enzymes and nutrient free radical quenchers. No viable cell can ever forget that oxygen is both friend and enemy.

THE HISTORY OF OXYGEN

Through most of geologic time, oxygen was not a problem. The earth's atmosphere contained none of this two-edged element. Atmospheric gases had been thrown into the sky by volcanoes and had leaked upwards through other geochemical processes—but oxygen was not among them.

Then several billion years ago, in the world's oceans and lakes, unicellular life began. These first organisms were anaerobic, like today's blue-green algae. They took their energy from the sun, synthesized it into sugar via fermentation—and released molecular oxygen as a useless by-product. Geologists can see this moment in the layered stone histories of the earth's activities. Suddenly the rocks streak red with rusted iron. Oxygen was on the loose.

It was only a century ago, however, in the late 1800s, that oxygen's destructive mechanics began to be understood. The first experiments revealed that free radicals derived from oxygen are responsible for the spoilage of fats and oils.[2] When butter goes rancid, oxy radicals are at work. Throughout most of the twentieth century, free radical research focused on food spoilage and on the role of free radicals in polymerization—especially in the creation of rubber and plastics.

Today, however, free radicals have moved front and center in the health sciences. They have turned out to be highly active in biological systems—and their exact mechanics are a matter of life and death.

WHAT IS A FREE RADICAL?

We have seen that a free radical is missing an electron—an electron it wants very badly. Why is this? The answer is found in the quantum mechanical structure of atoms and molecules.

In every atom, electrons inhabit shells, or orbits, around the nucleus. Each orbit has *sub-orbits*—known as *orbitals*. Like two-seater benches whirling around on a Ferris wheel, each circling orbital can accommodate two electrons. In fact, each orbital *prefers* to have two electrons. The trouble begins if an orbital (in an atom's outer orbit) has only one electron in it. This situation creates an intense thirst to match the unpaired electron with another one. Such an unstable and reactive atom (or molecule) is called a free radical—it has one or more unpaired electrons in outer shell orbitals.[3]

The situation is more complicated than it seems, since not all electrons will satisfy this free radical thirst. This is because not all electrons are equal. There are two fundamental types of electrons—defined by a quality that physicists call *spin*.

An electron's "spin" is typical of the Alice in Wonderland, sub-atomic world. Physicists know that electrons don't really spin; they know, in fact, that electrons aren't really solid particles at all. Rather, in the latest quantum mechanical field theories, electrons (and all other sub-atomic "particles") are understood to be *wave forms*—localized waves, or wave packets, fluctuating in an underlying non-material field (see Chapter Seven for more details).

Yet electrons do have a shadowy quantum mechanical quality that cannot be known precisely, but that resembles spin when described mathematically—so physicists use the word. Electrons display two types of spin. If a top is spinning, it may appear from above to be turning clockwise. When it is inverted, however, it will appear from the same vantage point to be turning counter-clockwise. Physicists refer to this difference as *spin up* or *spin down*.

For free radicals, the payoff is this: Two electrons nestled in a single orbital cannot be spinning the same way. Just as opposite electromagnetic charges attract and like charges repel, so opposite spins attract and like spins repel. In a free radical, an electron occupies an orbital by itself, yearning for its mate of opposite spin.

BIOCHEMICAL BAD BOYS

A free radical is intrinsically unstable, highly reactive with other atoms and molecules in the vicinity, and, for these reasons, short-lived.[4] These "biochemical bad boys," as an official publication of the National Institutes of Health calls them, cause systematic damage in every cell of the body.[5]

Superoxide. Known as the master oxygen radical, superoxide is often the first formed. Superoxide is molecular oxygen (O_2) which has grabbed an extra electron ($O_2^\bullet$). It can do damage on its own and it also breaks down spontaneously into hydrogen peroxide, then interacts with this offspring to produce the hydroxy radical.

Hydroxy radical. This is by far the most destructive free radical. It is one part oxygen and one part hydrogen ($OH^\bullet$) and it is the strongest oxidant known, the most powerful extractor of electrons.[6] The hydroxy radical is so wildly reactive that it typically lasts less than 0.000000001 seconds. It can incapacitate nearly anything it touches, including cell membrane lipids, large enzyme complexes, vitamin C, and DNA.[7] The unpaired electron in the hydroxy radical is extra, in terms of what OH by itself needs for internal stability. If the hydroxy radical ($OH^\bullet$) can't find a matching electron, it passes the extra electron on to another OH. With unimaginable speed, the electron zooms from OH to OH until it finds one close enough to a vulnerable molecule to cause a destructive reaction.[8] The hydroxy radical thus operates like a bucket brigade to spread destruction throughout the cell.

Lipid peroxy radical. This free radical is formed when the fatty molecules in cell membranes are attacked. When an electron is stolen from a membrane *lipid* (the biochemical term for fat), the lipid peroxy radical is produced. It is relatively large and has an immensely long half-life by free radical standards—seven seconds. We will soon review the damage this free radical creates as it first chain-reacts and then disintegrates.

Singlet oxygen. There are three *reactive oxygen species* (ROS) which are not technically free radicals, but are nonetheless highly reactive. Singlet oxygen is one of these reactive oxygen species, but it is relatively rare in living systems—usually a passing phase as oxygen shifts its shape from one damaging guise to another.[9]

Hydrogen peroxide. Hydrogen peroxide is an ROS which can persist indefinitely. It is also highly mobile; it can penetrate a cell membrane from the outside to do damage within. It can touch off peroxy chain reactions in the cell membrane, and will slowly degrade many biological molecules. At low concentrations it is not deadly to a cell, but by reacting with superoxide or metal ions, it gives birth to the lethal hydroxy radical.

Hypochlorous acid. Ordinarily formed when immune system cells go on the attack against outside invaders (see details below), hypochlorous acid is a brutally destructive combination of hydrogen peroxide and chlorine. Hypochlorous acid (a variety of which powers chlorine bleach) is particularly corrosive to proteins and their constituent parts (amino acids), as well as to the nucleotide bases that make up the DNA code.

WHY OXYGEN STARTS IT ALL

It is not a pretty line-up. And the common denominator is oxygen. But why? Compared with every other compound in a living system (except for some of its own oxy radical off-spring), oxygen has the greatest need for electrons. What are the properties of oxygen that give it such a ravenous electron hunger?

The answer lies in a quantum mechanical quirk in oxygen's structure. An oxygen atom has six electrons in its outer shell, a shell that can accept eight electrons total. One might expect that these six electrons would pair up two by two, leaving one empty orbital. If this were the case, the oxygen atom would still have a reasonably strong desire to pick up an additional pair of electrons to fill the last orbital in its outer shell. All atoms would rather have their outer shell full.

But oxygen is not a common case. Only four of its outer shell electrons pair off two by two. The last two electrons can't get together. They are both spin up. They repel each other and must occupy separate orbitals, alone and unpaired. Oxygen thus has *two* unpaired electrons—and its drive for additional electrons is thus uncommonly great. In a sense, in fact, oxygen is a free radical twice over. In discussions of free radicals an oxygen atom is frequently written •O•.

When two oxygen atoms combine into molecular oxygen, the same thing happens. The oxygen molecule ends up with two spin up electrons alone in two outer orbitals (molecules as a whole can have orbits and orbitals just like atoms).[10] Both of these electrons are hungry for a mate. This electron hunger makes molecular oxygen decidedly unstable. Like a single atom of oxygen, the oxygen molecule is, to a significant degree, a double-barreled free radical—what biochemists call a di-radical, or bi-radical.[11]

The net result: Oxygen is dangerous to our health. And many natural processes in the body transform oxygen into the even more dangerous oxy radicals and ROS. This chapter describes some of the most prolific of those processes:

1. The energy-producing mechanisms in every cell.

2. The desperate battles fought by the immune system.

3. The injury caused by chemicals and other pollution.

4. The self-destruction produced by mental and physical stress.

All of these produce free radicals. All damage our health.

TOXIC WASTE IN THE ENERGY PLANTS

The cell's energy system inadvertently operates as the most fundamental free radical factory in the body. Every cell has many powerhouses, known as *mitochondria*, which generate 90% of the energy used in the cell. In these organelles, glucose is burned in a controlled reaction—and free radicals and ROS are created as toxic waste. Nothing helps explain the intimate connection between oxygen-based life and oxygen-based death more precisely than these energy-producing processes.[12]

A large corporation that manufactures, say, computers, might buy and incorporate a smaller business that specializes in making computer power supplies. Some billions of years ago small, single-celled organisms apparently made a similar incorporation. They came upon other, smaller cells that had learned to use oxygen to generate vast amounts of energy from glucose. The large cells took in the smaller ones and put them to use.

Today, most biochemists believe, every cell in the human body is a descendant from those early combinations. The power-generating mitochondria that populate our cells still maintain many signs of being a separate, symbiotic life form—they have their own DNA and the ability to divide and replicate within the larger cell. From this partnership, the larger cell gains energy, while the mitochondria gain a warm, relatively safe home with an abundant food supply.

Mitochondria are mobile and very active within the cell, moving to the sites where energy is needed most and replicating rapidly when energy needs are great. Muscle cells and brain cells especially are densely packed with these small, semi-independent energy plants.

Mitochondria consist largely of a double layer of membrane—an outer, roughly elliptical membrane and an inner membrane that folds back on itself accordion-style and stuffs the outer membrane as full as possible. For the mitochondria, this inner membrane functions as a work surface. Packed densely all over this rippling inner membrane are complex electron processors, the active, energy-creating sites. Each processor is, in round numbers, only one-millionth of an inch wide and 0.3-millionths of an inch thick. In molecular terms, however, they are gigantic, packing together molecules boasting a molecular weight of 500,000 and more. (Molecular weight is the sum of all the atomic weights involved; the touchstone atomic weight is carbon's: 12.) There are roughly 100,000 of these molecular energy plants situated on the inner membrane of every mitochondrion. Each consists of 15 to 20 massive enzymes embedded in precise sequence directly into the membrane itself, held in place by the lipid membrane molecules.

These energy-creating complexes begin their work when electrons are deposited into the front end of the enzyme sequence. The first enzyme has a quantum mechanical need for an electron at its active site, and therefore accepts the electron. However, the electron hunger of this first enzyme is not as great as the hunger of the second enzyme. As the random heat motion of cell molecules causes the enzymes to turn and twist in place, the second enzyme eventually faces the newly acquired electron in the first. Instantly, it steals that electron away.

Down through the entire line-up of enzymes, moreover, each additional enzyme has a greater need for electrons than the previous one. As the enzymes turn and twist, the electron is pulled inexorably down the chain (called the *electron transport chain*) like a marble through the chutes and trap doors of a Rube Goldberg device. In ways that are not yet fully understood, this "downhill" flow of the electron is converted into molecules of adenosine triphosphate (ATP), which store energy for use in the cell. Like a waterfall turning a turbine to create electricity, the flow of electrons creates ATP.

At the bottom of the chain, with its ominous electron hunger, oxygen waits to snatch up electrons at the end of their run. Without oxygen, in fact, the whole chain wouldn't operate. Oxygen pulls the electrons off the last enzyme. If it didn't, the last enzyme would remain full and would not pull electrons from the next enzyme up the chain. Choked off at the bottom, the chain would back up and cease to flow.

This electron transport chain is an astonishingly efficient energy plant. Without it, the cell can still take a glucose molecule (a simple row of six linked carbon atoms edged with 14 hydrogens) and split it once. This is an anaerobic process (*glycolysis*) and yields two molecules of ATP. However, two ATP molecules from one glucose molecule is a pitifully small yield. The mitochondria can do much better than that. First, they strip all the hydrogen atoms off the split glucose molecules. Then they deposit the electrons from these hydrogen atoms into the electron transport chain. By the time all the electrons from a single glucose molecule have run down the chain, 36 more ATP molecules have been created. Biochemists believe this system recovers anywhere from 50% to 80% of the available energy (a gasoline engine, in comparison, is good for only about 10% recovery).

THE PRICE OF ENERGY

The price of this efficiency, however, is the presence of oxygen. With electrons loose, rolling down the chain, and oxygen lurking about, hungry for electrons, the chance of mishap is high.[13] At first glance, it might seem the greatest danger is at the end of the chain, where oxygen takes its appointed role as the final electron acceptor. This danger, however, has been taken into account. The final enzyme conglomerate in the chain, known as *cytochrome oxidase*, leaves nothing to chance. First, it splits molecular oxygen into two oxygen atoms, taking a firm grip on both. Then it runs both atoms through a sequence of reactions in which it essentially inserts two hydrogen atoms into each captive oxygen. At the end, it releases two water molecules (H_2O) into the aqueous fluid suffusing the cell. The oxygen has been safely imprisoned in the water molecule, which is the most stable oxygen compound. In the water molecule, oxygen's dual electron hunger has been satisfied by sharing one electron from each hydrogen. It holds on to these shared electrons with such avidity that no other atom can take them away.[14]

The truth is, however, oxygen does not take a number and wait patiently in line at the end of the transport chain. Oxygen is everywhere—in the chinks between major enzyme conglomerates, at the head of the chain, and in the fluid on both sides of the membrane where transport molecules are carrying electrons to the chain. Some scientists isolate two spots as most perilous. One is the head of the chain, known as the *Q reductase* enzyme grouping, where carrier molecules first drop off loose electrons. Because this initial enzyme has the least electron hunger of any in the chain, oxygen can successfully compete for electrons before they get started down the chain.[15]

Another especially vulnerable spot is the *ubiquinone* complex, a smaller series of enzymes in the middle of the chain.

Ubiquinone is completely enclosed in the lipid in the middle of the membrane. Oxygen, unfortunately, is soluble in lipid. It has direct access to the ubiquinone complex. Some scientists believe, in fact, that in the ubiquinone complex, oxygen is taken up and the superoxide free radical created—as a routine and integral part of the larger electron transport process.[16]

The best estimates are that 98% or more of the electrons go down the transport chain and get deposited into water molecules without mishap. One or two percent, however, go astray.[17] Of this remnant, most are initially taken up by oxygen (O_2) to create superoxide ($O_2^\bullet$), the master free radical, which soon gives rise to other free radicals and ROS.

THE END OF ENERGY

It's true the mitochondria are armed against these free radical dangers (see Chapter Four). Like police on patrol in a high-crime neighborhood, several enzyme systems that scavenge free radicals populate the mitochondria in high numbers.

But foolproof defense is difficult to ensure. Research has made it clear that oxy radicals produced in the mitochondria escape the defense systems to do serious long-term damage. In fact, the damage caused by such oxy radicals has been highlighted by one of biology's most striking statistics: There are strict energy-production limits on the lifetime of each animal species. Each species has, on the average, only a set number of calories it can burn in its lifetime. Put another way, the rate of aging in any species is generally proportional to the metabolic rate of that species. The faster the metabolic rate, the shorter the life span.

It has long puzzled researchers why such limitations should exist. Now the free radical paradigm has provided an explanation. The more quickly you use oxygen to burn glucose, the more quickly you produce oxy radicals and ROS as toxic waste. Burning calories is ultimately a self-limiting process.[18]

Research at the National Institute of Aging (NIA) has tied this to free radical damage. This work has demonstrated that some mammals can burn many more calories per pound of body weight than others. Mice and gerbils, for instance, are given an average life allotment of 200,000 calories per gram of body weight. When they have burned that many calories, on the average, their lives end. Non-human primates, on the other hand, have double the allotment, 400,000 calories per gram, and humans get double that again, roughly 800,000 calories per gram.[19]

When you fuel up your car and drive down the road, friction causes a certain amount of damage in the engine. The more gasoline you burn (and the more miles you drive), the more damage the friction causes. After a certain accumulation of damage, the engine dies. In a similar way, the more energy the body burns, the more free radicals are created—and free radicals cause friction in the physiology.

Why can humans burn four times more calories and thus, theoretically, produce four times more oxy radicals than lower mammals before succumbing to the inevitable damage? Dr. Richard Cutler of the NIA has demonstrated that short-lived species have low levels of anti-oxidants in comparison to their average metabolic rate. Long-lived species in general have high levels of anti-oxidants, and humans have the highest. Apparently, human beings can run their metabolic equipment longer because they detoxify free radicals more efficiently.[20]

The body burns calories by stripping electrons off glucose molecules and moving them down the electron transport chain to oxygen. Apparently, it is only possible to move so many electrons down that chain. Each of those electrons is playing Russian roulette with the omni-present oxygen. A reasonably steady percentage go awry, gobbled up as part of free radical generation. A reasonably steady percentage of those free radicals apparently slip by the body's defenses as well and create their damage.[21]

The scale of the problem defies comprehension. There are trillions of cells in the body, each with hundreds, sometimes thousands of mitochondria, each of which in turn may have more than 100,000 electron transport chains. In every mitochondrion, all the time, an unimaginable number of electrons are tumbling down these chains. In every mitochondrion, all the time, a steady percentage of these electrons are being diverted to create free radicals. Along with the energy that mitochondria give to their host cell, they also bequeath self-destruction through the toxic waste we call oxy radicals and ROS.

TOXIC WASTE FROM THE IMMUNE SYSTEM

As mentioned in Chapter One, there is another important physiological system that creates free radicals in large numbers. This problem is not so constant, nor so inexorable as in the mitochondria. In sudden emergencies, however, the damage can be much more acute. When microbes invade the body, fast-reacting cells in the immune system charge to the scene, spewing out the most destructive oxy radicals and ROS. The result is often severe collateral damage to cells in the surrounding area. The immune system can damage what it is meant to protect.

The body needs a powerful immune system, of course. The debt we owe to a healthy immune system has been demonstrated all too obviously by the devastating results of AIDS (*acquired immunodeficiency syndrome*)—which systematically cripples the immune system and leaves the body defenseless in the face of ever-present infectious microbes.

The interior of a warm-blooded body is well-protected and well-nourished—ideal not only for its own cells but also for many invaders. The two most common types of interloper are bacteria and viruses—and the damaging varieties must be stopped to maintain good health.

To cope with these threats, the immune system has developed a multitudinous and richly varied set of weapons. In a book focused on free radicals, however, it is only necessary to understand the operation of the immune system's first line of defense—its rapid deployment forces—the white blood cells which most quickly respond to signs of an invader.

When bacteria or viruses first enter the body, cells in the local area begin to be damaged. These cells emit a chemical call for help. When the lipid molecules in cell membranes are damaged, these damaged molecules (known as *lipid peroxides*) trigger a particular set of chemical reactions known as the *arachidonic acid pathway*. The result is certain biochemicals— *leukotrienes* and *prostaglandins*—which are attractive to particular immune system cells. These attractor biochemicals diffuse away from the site of injury through blood vessels and intercellular spaces. Like heat-seeking missiles, the white blood cells spontaneously move toward increasing concentrations of these attractor chemicals. The process is known as *chemotaxis*.

The first cell to arrive is usually the *neutrophil*. Neutrophils are small and live only a few days. The bone marrow of a healthy human being creates as many as 100 billion neutrophils every day to maintain a sufficient supply. Roughly half of these circulate in the blood and half cling to artery walls. Normally, neutrophils are in the idle mode, using anaerobic glycolysis to burn as little energy as possible. When they detect one of the alarm chemicals emitted by damaged cells, however, chemotaxis takes them rapidly to the area under attack. Their small size allows them to slip easily through pores in the artery walls and slide through intercellular spaces until they reach the battleground—usually within minutes. Then they show their true nature.

First they ingest an invader. Then they inhale fifty times more oxygen than they usually contain—an action known as the *respiratory burst*—and use the oxygen to generate a toxic shower of oxy radicals and ROS.[22] Superoxide is the first oxy radical produced. It partially decomposes into hydrogen peroxide and then interacts with this offspring to create the hydroxy radical. High concentrations of chloride ion are also generated, and chloride reacts with hydrogen peroxide to create protein-eating hypochlorous acid.[23] The neutrophils spray this lethal combination on the captured invader. Taking no chances, the neutrophil also unloads large quantities of digestive enzymes from its lysosomes to break the invaders' molecules down.

The battle can be fierce. Trapped bacteria can squirm and writhe, all the while pouring out toxins, before succumbing to the neutrophil's lethal shower. The neutrophil is a worthy warrior—arriving first, and with the most fire power[24]—and after one victory, it moves right on to another battle, annihilating an average of 25 enemies before finally giving in to accumulated injury.

Neutrophils carry on the battle alone for the first several hours. Then reinforcements begin to arrive. These are known as monocytes (in their ordinary guise). Rather than circulating in the blood stream, monocytes are usually stationed permanently in particular tissues. They move within that area using an ameboid style of motion—extruding an arm in one direction, taking hold on a handy surface, then pulling the main body up to join. It's not a speedy process. Though they are sometimes relatively close to the site of invasion, they can still take several hours to arrive on the scene. But monocytes make up for their delayed arrival at the battleground with an awesome transformer trick. When faced with invaders, they suddenly enlarge many times over. All immune cells that do direct battle with external pathogens are known as *phagocytes* ("eaters of cells"); in its new giant form the monocyte is known as a *macrophage* ("big eater").

Normally, macrophages act as the body's janitors—cleaning up dead cells, oxidized molecules, cancerous cells, and low concentrations of infectious agents. Unlike neutrophils, they can live for months, even years, tending their housekeeping tasks. In a major invasion, however, they also show their true colors. Although their respiratory burst is only one-quarter as intense as that of neutrophils, their staying power is much greater.[25] They reach out long arms, grab up bacteria and viruses on the sticky surface, then engulf them and shower them with oxy radicals, ROS, and digestive enzymes—keeping up the fight through successful encounters with 100 or more opponents. Macrophages also act as scouts in a long-term fight, identifying enemy organisms, processing them, and presenting them to a third wave of immune system cells. The macrophages also clean up dead neutrophils, dead or damaged cells, and other debris on the battlefield.

While fighting, macrophages also release a biochemical known as interleukin-1, which travels to a cluster of neurons in the brain's hypothalamus. As a result, the body increases its level of internal heat (it "runs a fever"). As the heat increases, most of the bacteria become less mobile and they slow their rate of reproduction. By sending interleukin-1 to the hypothalamus, macrophages tip the scales in their favor.[26]

THE COST OF DEFENSE

We literally owe our lives to neutrophils, macrophages, and other specialized cells in the immune system. But it must be said that the use of high-powered weaponry by these defense forces is not always under ideal control. In fact, excess oxy radicals and ROS spilled into the environment by the hard-pressed neutrophils and macrophages can result in widespread cell damage.[27]

The entire syndrome by which these first defenders take on an enemy is known as the *inflammatory response*. The first damaged cells in a given area not only release chemotactic cries for assistance, they also emit other substances which expand capillaries in the local region, drawing in more blood—including white blood cells. The battle, with its consequent damage to local cells, increases the inflammation. For a brief time, as an emergency measure, this inflammatory response is more useful than damaging. (Elderly people, for example, frequently have a diminished capacity for the inflammatory response, and this produces a diminished capacity for fighting infections.)

But the inflammatory response has an unfortunate tendency to feed on itself. Like an atomic reactor accelerating out of control, the first inflammatory interactions beget later ones in a cycle that is hard to break. If the inflammation lasts too long, the collateral damage becomes too great. The culprits in this excessive inflammation are oxy radicals and ROS.

In the first place, neutrophils, macrophages, and other phagocytes create their death-dealing oxygen compounds in enzymatic sites embedded in their outer cell membranes. Some of these oxy radicals and ROS go inward, toward invaders which have been engulfed and trapped within the phagocyte. But by manufacturing the oxy radicals and ROS in their outer membrane, the phagocytes can easily spill large quantities into the surrounding environment.[28] This may not be just an error. A cleaner system would keep all the dangerous oxygen compounds within the phagocyte, concentrated on the captured invader—but the phagocytes may be fighting on two fronts at once. By releasing destructive hydroxy radicals and hypochlorous acid into the environment, they can weaken prospective combatants even as they focus on the foe in hand. In a desperate struggle, this can turn the tide.

In any event, whether they are leaked during battle or result from the eventual death and disintegration of phagocytes, a wide range of destructive oxy radicals and ROS flood the environment as an inevitable by-product of the inflammatory reaction.[29] The first problem caused by such an excessive use of free radicals is often damage to the immune system cells themselves. They live and die by the free radical sword. Without strong anti-oxidant protection, their effectiveness in a fight has been shown to be much weaker.[30]

Moreover, free radicals can stimulate a vicious cycle, as damage begets more damage, driving the inflammatory reaction out of control. High concentrations of the hydroxy radical, for example, can seriously damage the lipid membranes of nearby cells, creating lipid peroxide. These lipid peroxide molecules stimulate the production of leukotrienes and prostaglandins, the emergency chemicals which float off into intercellular spaces and the blood stream, acting as chemotactic beacons to draw in more phagocytes.

The new phagocytes do even more damage, and the cycle feeds on itself. What's worse, the arachidonic acid reactions that create these chemotactic chemical messengers also generate more free radicals as a toxic by-product, adding to the molecular chaos. In addition, superoxide interacts with normally benign molecules floating loose in the blood plasma to create even more chemotaxis.[31]

Finally, after the phagocytes release protease and other powerful digestive enzymes as part of their destructive weaponry, they also release other enzymes which act to inhibit the digestive enzymes and keep their damage under control. These inhibiting enzymes, however, are attacked by both the hydroxy radical and hypochlorous acid. The brake is released, and the digestive enzymes can attack surrounding cells.[32]

In this self-propelled destruction, the greatest immediate damage is done by hydroxy radicals and hypochlorous acid. However, superoxide and hydrogen peroxide both last longer—in fact, hydrogen peroxide can last indefinitely if it doesn't react with another molecule. Both of these can also penetrate cell membranes and create damage *inside* neighboring cells. What's more, N-chloroamine, another electron-hungry compound created during the respiratory burst, has a half-life of 18 hours. It breaks down alpha-1-protease inhibitor, increasing the damage done by digestive enzymes, and it can diffuse over long distances in its relatively long lifetime to initiate other types of damage.[33]

It thus appears that oxy radicals and ROS are the major factor in pushing the inflammatory reaction out of control. This has been confirmed in a long series of experiments and clinical trials in which various anti-oxidant substances have been shown to suppress the inflammatory reaction both in the laboratory and in human subjects.[34] As we will see in the next chapter, chronic inflammation can produce many diseases, from rheumatoid arthritis to cancer. The immune system's use of free radical weaponry can get out of hand, with serious short-term and long-term effects.

POLLUTION AND OTHER EXTERNAL CAUSES

Those of us who live in the twentieth century face another serious free radical threat. Although the last hundred years or so have often been called the Industrial Age, they might just as easily have been called the Age of Chemicals. We have unraveled many secrets of the molecule and learned to manipulate molecular bonding mechanisms to create exotic new compounds. These new chemicals have given us automobile tires, fertilizers and pesticides, and anti-cancer drugs. But they have also given us a wide range of diseases—by infusing our environment with an ever-rising level of toxic substances, many of them operating through free radical mechanisms. Even a brief list of well-publicized offenders is a source of dismay:

Toxins

    Carbon tetrachloride

    Paraquat

    Benzo(a)pyrene

    Aniline dyes

    Toluene

Drugs

    Adriamycin

    Bleomycin

    Mitomycin C

    Nitrofurantoin

    Chlorpromazine

Air Pollution

    Primary sources

        Carbon monoxide

        Nitric oxide

        Unburned hydrocarbons

    Secondary sources

        Ozone

        Nitrogen dioxide

        Aldehydes

        Alkyl nitrates

Other environmental sources of free radicals include:

- Alcohol
- Tobacco smoke
- Smoked and barbecued food
- Peroxidized fats in meat and aged cheeses
- Radiation

It must be said that even sunlight, a personal pleasure and in many ways healthful, also creates free radicals in the skin. That's why ladies in the ante-bellum south always walked under parasols. That's why sun worshippers look old before their time. Sun-generated free radicals cross-link the protein in the skin's collagen, causing stiffness and wrinkles.[35]

What this all means is that the human physiology, challenged already by free radicals from within, must cope with an increasing flood from outside.

Environmental toxins: Among the poisonous chemicals which appear to create their damage through free radical mechanisms are carbon tetrachloride (used in fire extinguishers and as an industrial solvent; it breaks down into the free radical carbon trichloride to cause severe liver damage), paraquat (a herbicide known to destroy the DNA in plant cells; it causes severe lung damage through cross-linking of proteins),[36] and adriamycin (an anti-cancer drug that can cause fatal heart damage).[37]

Many of the most potent environmental toxins—including a large number of pesticides, herbicides, industrial chemicals, and drugs—appear to follow similar pathways in the body when ingested. They are first shipped to "detox" units available in every cell. Known as *cytochrome P-450*, these detoxification complexes are another example of electron transport chains. They are embedded in folded membranes known as the *endoplasmic reticulum*, located near the cell nucleus.[38]

The problem is that there are many types of cytochrome P-450 (also known as the *mixed function oxidase system*), probably hundreds of variations. Most do their job well—but not all. Some unfortunately create hydrogen peroxide or superoxide as a standard by-product of their operation. Even worse, some, while trying to detoxify an ingested chemical, transform it into a particularly brutal type of free radical—one that can steal an electron, pass it off to oxygen, steal another electron, make another pass, and keep it up indefinitely (a process known as *redox cycling*). The original molecule may have been only mildly toxic, or even inert. The transformed molecule is a free radical factory.[39]

These free radical-creating molecules are at home within the lipid membranes that house electron transport chains. Many scientists believe these transformed molecules insert themselves into a local electron transport chain and continuously steal electrons running down the chain.[40] One of the cell's most ingenious mechanisms is thus twisted into an assembly line of self-destruction.[41]

Pharmaceuticals: Certain anti-cancer drugs appear to use a different mechanism. One end of the molecule attaches firmly to the DNA within the cancer cell, while the other end takes on iron and uses it for a cycling reaction that mass produces hydroxy radicals and other damaging oxygen species.[42] These oxy radicals damage the DNA, and the cancer cell dies.[43] This phenomenon suggests two things:

1. Cancer may originally be caused by free radical damage to the DNA.

2. Anti-cancer drugs may damage the DNA in healthy cells, producing new cancers. In fact, many anti-tumor drugs have been shown to cause new cancers.[44]

Vasodilating drugs cause free radical damage in yet a third way. By dilating blood vessels and causing a sudden increase in blood flow to various organs in the body, these drugs bring a sudden increase of oxygen to the cells involved. Free radicals rapidly damage both mitochondria and DNA.[45]

If the Industrial Age could be called the Age of Chemicals, it could also be called the Age of Free Radicals.

Air pollution: Unfortunately, we do not even need to eat or drink toxic chemicals to suffer physiological damage from externally caused free radicals. Simply breathing is often enough. When we breathe air polluted with emissions from gasoline engines, for example, we inhale prepackaged free radicals that can go to work immediately. The original by-products of combustion, such as carbon monoxide and nitric oxide, have negative effects by themselves. In the presence of sunlight and oxygen, moreover, these by-products are transformed into ozone and nitrogen dioxide, chemicals with the telltale unpaired electron. While ozone forms the life-protecting ozone layer high in the atmosphere and nitrogen dioxide is used as an industrial oxidant, research indicates that neither is among those gases which human beings should inhale. They peroxidize cell membranes and inactivate proteins, causing severe lung damage as a result.[46]

Tobacco smoke: Common habits can also be free radical sources. Tobacco smoke, for example, generates phenoxy free radicals by itself, and reacts in the body to create other free radicals. These free radicals damage cell membranes and cross-link proteins, leading to lung fibrosis and emphysema.

Alcohol: Alcohol is metabolized into the double free radical acetaldehyde, which can attack and cross-link macromolecules in the liver. Some researchers theorize that the metabolism of alcohol in the liver also creates excess electrons, leading to the creation of other free radicals.[47] Certainly, excess alcohol consumption produces fibrotic scarring and tissue death in the liver.[48]

Radiation: It is also true that electromagnetic radiation (including ultraviolet rays from the sun and radiation used in X-rays and cancer therapies) causes damage through the creation of free radicals. For example, one electron in a water molecule can absorb energy from external radiation. This excess energy excites the electron and kicks it out of its orbital and up to a higher orbit. The apparently safe water molecule thus becomes unstable. It breaks down (in a process called *hydrolysis*) to by-products that include the deadly hydroxy radical.[49] Thus, the danger posed by radiation can be great. Water molecules far outnumber all other molecules in the body put together; a process that can generate the hydroxy radical from water is extremely dangerous. Research has shown that radiation-induced hydroxy radicals can damage proteins, lipoproteins, and DNA, inhibit the process of mitosis (cell division), and kill cells outright.[50] In addition, it is well known that radiation therapy frequently creates new tumors while killing old ones.[51]

Processed foods: Finally, many processed foods—especially meats and aged cheeses—have lipid peroxide in them. Once ingested, the lipid peroxide can deteriorate further into free radicals and ROS, and take part in reactions that lead toward atherosclerosis (see Chapter Three).[52]

STRESS AND OXIDATIVE STRESS

In modern civilization, one other source of free radicals has a major effect on aging and disease. The free radical load is dangerously increased by the rigors of *stress*.

Medical experts have long known that stress resides not in the environment, but in our reaction to the environment. The stress syndrome is, in a sense, a psycho-physiological mistake—based on a biochemical apparatus that was set up to handle problems very different from the ones we face in modern urban life. The human system was built to deal with the short-term emergencies of prehistoric times—the hungry bears and flash floods our ancestors faced. The current reality, however, is usually slow-burn aggravation—the traffic jams and irate bosses that plague day-to-day existence.

The result of our reaction to these problems is neurochemical overkill. A loud horn or disapproving memo can trigger the system into a full-fledged *fight-or-flight* response. The adrenal and pituitary glands flood the system with hormones and the sympathetic branch of the autonomic nervous system mobilizes the body for defensive action. The system goes into its most excited state, ready for a fight or a full-speed escape. But in the modern world, there is often no way to discharge this extra energy and no defined end to the crisis. Instead, the physiology becomes hyper-aroused and stays that way for long periods. In fact, many people in modern society live most of their lives with the stress thermostat set much too high.

It has long been known that such constant stress can predispose people to many types of illness. The reason has only recently become clear: Constant stress generates a constant flow of free radicals. In the first place, the stress syndrome over-excites the body. High levels of cortisol in the bloodstream cause cells to shut down most of their normal maintenance activities and focus on energy creation. Even muscle tissue is broken down for use as fuel. The function of this reaction is to make the maximum possible energy available for fight or flight. That's why people under stress tend to pace up and down or go out to exercise and "work it off."

This kind of hyperactivity—the jitters—is more than an inconvenience. Such extra energy creation means a speedup in the mitochondrial electron transport chain—with an automatic increase in free radical creation. A fast-moving chain gives oxygen more target electrons on the move down the chain. Some researchers also feel that excess speed makes the chain operation itself sloppier, with a higher percentage of electrons escaping.[53]

Cortisol and other stress-related chemicals cause further problems. For example, both cortisol and the catecholamines —including epinephrine and norepinephrine—lead to the creation of leukotrienes and thromboxanes. This chemical pathway systematically produces free radicals as toxic waste.[54] Even worse, catecholamines themselves break down into free radicals, and some into free radical factories—redox cycling molecules that can insert themselves into electron transport chains and hand off electrons to oxygen.[55]

In several potent ways, therefore, stress causes the body to produce its own toxic substances. In fact, some researchers now suggest that stress should be given a new definition:

Biological stress is that which accelerates the production of oxy radicals and ROS in human cells and tissues.[56]

Stress translates into oxidative stress.

MEASURING YOUR FREE RADICAL LOAD

Researchers have catalogued the many processes that produce free radicals—including the mitochondrial energy plants, the rapid reaction forces of the immune system, external pollutants and the body's reaction to them, and the self-toxicity produced by stress. They have speculated that, if free radical creation outstrips the body's defenses, then progressive damage inevitably results.

It is this disequilibrium, or free radical *overhang*, that provides the most precise definition of oxidative stress.[57] In this view, oxidative stress—a constant preponderance of free radicals over natural defenses—amounts to a continual metabolic friction in oxygen-breathing organisms.[58] Such constant oxidative friction wears the body down three ways:

1. It weakens the immune system defenses against infectious disease.

2. It produces degenerative disease.

3. It stimulates the systematic physiological deterioration called aging.[59]

Because of the central importance of oxidative stress, some researchers have suggested that for every patient with any disease, the total load of oxidative stress should be assessed. They recommend a number of blood tests for this purpose: measurements of (1) lipid peroxide levels, (2) the ratio of vitamin C to oxidized vitamin C (oxidized vitamin C has already encountered a free radical), and (3) the level of an anti-oxidant enzyme (glutathione peroxidase) in red blood cells.[60]

By taking these measurements—to roughly assess the current levels of oxidative damage being done by free radicals—

medical authorities would accomplish at least two things. First, they would have a new measure of the severity of any given illness; if ongoing free radical damage were high, then regardless of current symptoms, the situation might be troublesome. Second, they would have a signal for the introduction of generalized approaches to reduce oxidative stress.

Regardless of what else is done to deal with the specific illness, it would always be useful to reduce the free radical overhang. By reducing the total load of oxidative stress, the physiology as a whole would be strengthened. Recovery from any specific illness would theoretically be enhanced.

In fact, it is theoretically possible to use such tests of oxidative stress on people who are currently healthy. You may feel fine, but if free radicals have even a slight advantage over your body's defenses, then metabolic friction is taking place—inevitably and continually. The body is getting older. The seeds are being sown for future disease.

As the tests become more refined, it may be possible to assess the balance point for oxidative stress. Each person would have an ongoing feedback mechanism to indicate if more anti-oxidant approaches are necessary. There may be no way to avoid air pollution where you live, for example, but oxidative stress tests may someday be able to tell you when to increase your intake of anti-oxidants or your use of stress management programs to tip the physiological balance in your favor. Such tests would therefore be a means of continually assessing the success of preventive medicine programs. You would not have to wait 20 or 30 years to make sure you were doing enough to avoid cancer or heart disease. A simple blood test would keep you on track.

Without such attention to oxidative stress loads, the damage continues unabated. As we will see in the next chapter, medical scientists have now defined how accumulated free radical injury produces a wide array of specific diseases. It is a disconcerting tale with, fortunately, a happy ending.

Notes

1. Much of this chapter reviews basic aspects of molecular structure and activities in the cell—information available in any basic textbook on the subject. For lay readers interested in further detail, I recommend books from the *Scientific American* series: Atkins PW, *Atoms, Electrons, and Change* (Scientific American Library, New York, 1991); Atkins PW, *Molecules* (Scientific American Library, New York, 1987); de Duve C, *A Guided Tour of the Living Cell, Volumes 1 & 2* (Scientific American Library, New York, 1984). For more substance, an excellent university textbook, well organized and clearly written, is: Alberts B, et al, *Molecular Biology of the Cell* (Garland Publishing, Inc., New York, 1983)

2. Dormandy T, *Lancet* 2(1969): 684-8

3. Southorn P, Powis G, *Mayo Clin Proc* 63(1988): 381-9

4. Brown W, *Introduction to Organic Chemistry* (Williard Grant Press, Boston, 1982), p. 98

5. Hooper C, *J NIH Res* 1(1989): 101-6. This selection gives a readable introduction to the important free radicals and ROS.

6. Piette LH, "Ageing and Cancer: A Common Free Radical Mechanism?" in *Interrelationship Among Aging, Cancer, and Differentiation*, Pullman B, et al, eds. (D. Reidel Publishing Company, 1985), pp. 301-12

7. Hooper, *J NIH* (see note 5)

8. Elizabeth Dimock, Biochemist, Maharishi International University, personal communication (July 1992)

9. Richards RT, Sharma HM, *Ind J Clin Prac* 2(1991): 15-26

10. Dimock (see note 8)

11. Dormandy T, *Lancet* 2(1969): 684-8; Demopoulos HB, et al, *Env Pathol Toxicol* 3(1980): 272-303

12. For the non-specialist, a good description of mitochondria and energy production can be found in Christian de Duve's book, *A Guided Tour of the Living Cell* (See note 1), pp. 148-66. A more thorough analysis is in *Molecular Biology of the Cell*, Alberts B, et al (see note 1). A specific free radical analysis of the mitochondrial electron transport chain is found in *Current Concepts: Oxygen-Derived Radicals and Their Metabolites: Relationship to Tissue Injury*, Fantone JC, Ward PA (The Upjohn Company, Kalamazoo, 1985). The author is also indebted to molecular biologist John Fagan at Maharishi International University for insights into recent research on the topic.

13. Niwa Y, Tsutsui D, *Saishinigaku* (Japan) 38(1983): 1450-8

14. Bendich A, "Antioxidant Nutrients and Immune Functions" in *Antioxidant Nutrients and Immune Functions,* Bendich A, et al, eds. (Plenum Press, New York, 1990), pp. 1-12; McCord J, *Surgery* 94(1983): 412-4

15. Forman HJ, Boveris A, "Superoxide Radical and Hydrogen Peroxide in Mitochondria" in *Free Radicals in Biology, Vol. 5,* Pryor WA, ed. (Academic Press, New York, 1982), pp. 65-90

16. Fantone, *Current* (see note 12), pp. 9-10

17. Forman , "Superoxide" (see note 15)

18. Cutler RG, *Am J Clin Nutr* 53(1991): 373S-9S

19. Cutler RG, *Gerontol* 25(1979): 69-86

20. Cutler, *Am* (see note 18)

21. Ibid

22. Babior BM, "The Role of Active Oxygen in Microbial Killing by Phagocytes" in *Pathology of Oxygen,* Autor AP, ed. (Academic Press, New York, 1982), pp. 45-58; Bendich, "Antioxidant" (see note 14)

23. Fantone, *Current* (see note 12), p. 6-7; Halliwell B, *Cell Biol Int Repts* 6(1982): 529-42

24. Tsuda H, et al, *J Biochem* 95(1984): 1237-45

25. Ibid

26. Faith RE, et al, "Interactions Between the Immune System and the Nervous System" in *Stress and Immunity,* Plotnikoff N, et al, eds. (CRC Press, Boca Raton, 1991) pp. 287-304

27. Boxer L, "The Role of Antioxidants in Modulating Neutrophil Functional Responses" in *Antioxidant Nutrients and Immune Functions,* Bendich A, et al, eds. (Plenum Press, New York, 1990), pp. 19-33

28. Fantone, *Current* (see note 12), p. 13; Miyachi Y, et al, *Arch Dermatol Res* 277(1985): 288-92

29. Fridovich I, "Superoxide Dismutase in Biology and Medicine" in *Pathology of Oxygen,* Autor AP, ed. (Academic Press, New York, 1982), pp. 1-19; Halliwell, *Cell* (see note 23)

30. Levine SA, Kidd PM, *Antioxidant Adaptation: Its Role in Free Radical Pathology* (Biocurrents Division, Allergy Research Group, San Leandro, 1986), p. 296

31. Fridovich I, "Superoxide" (see note 29)

32. Fantone, *Current* (see note 12), p. 28

33. Weiss SJ, et al, *Science* 222(1983): 625-8

34. Levine SA, *Int J Biosocial Res* 4(1983): Part One 51-4, Part Two 102-5; Warso MA, Lands WEM, *British Med Bull* 39(1983): 277-80; Bryant

RW, et al, *J Biol Chem* 257(1982): 14937-43; Metz SA, *Med Clin N Am* 65(Symposium Issue)(1981): 713-57; Huber W, Menander-Huber KB, *Clinics in Rheum Dis* 6(1980): 465-98

35. Richards, *Indian* (see note 9); Fantone, *Current* (see note 12), p. 38

36. Fisher HK, et al, *Ann Intern Med* 75(1971): 731-6

37. Southorn P, Powis G, *Mayo Clin Proc* 63(1988): 390-408; Fantone, *Current* (see note 12), pp. 1-51

38. The author is indebted for details on cytochrome P-450 to John Fagan, Molecular Biologist, Maharishi International University, personal communication (August 1992)

39. Mason RP, Chignell CF, *Pharmacol Rev* 33(1982): 189-211; Mason RP, "Free Radical Intermediates in the Metabolism of Toxic Chemicals" in *Free Radicals in Biology, Vol 5*, Pryor WA, ed. (Academic Press, New York, 1982), pp. 161-222

40. Ernster L, et al, "Microsomal Lipid Peroxidation: Mechanism and Some Biomedical Implications" in *Lipid Peroxides in Biology and Medicine*, Yagi K, ed. (Academic Press, New York, 1982), pp. 55-79; Bachur NR, et al, *Proc Natl Acad Sci USA* 76(1979): 954-7; Powis G, et al, *Mol Pharmacol* 20(1981): 387-94; Bachur NR, et al, *Cancer Res* 38(1978): 1745-50; Schenkman JB, et al, *Mol Pharmacol* 15(1979): 428-38; Nelson SD, et al, *Biochem Biophys Res Comm* 70(1976): 1157-65

41. Levine, *Antioxidant* (see note 30), p. 35

42. Burger RM, et al, *Life Sci* 28(1981): 715-27; Lin PS, et al, *Cancer* 46(1980): 2360-4

43. Piette, "Ageing" (see note 6); Peto R, et al, *Nature* 290(1980): 201

44. Ibid

45. Fackelmann KA, *Science News* 140(1991): 214-5

46. Mustafa MG, Tierney DF, *Am Rev Respir Dis* 118(1978): 1061-90

47. Cotran RS, et al, eds., *Robbins Pathologic Basis of Disease* (W.B. Saunders Co., Philadelphia, 1989), pp. 490-2, 944-9

48. Ibid

49. Greenstock CL, *Rad Res* 86(1981): 196-211

50. Bielski BHJ, Gabicki JM, "Application of Radiation Chemistry to Biology" in *Free Radicals in Biology, Vol. 3*, Pryor WA, ed. (Academic Press Inc., New York, 1977), pp. 1-51

51. Richards, *Indian* (see note 9)

52. Yagi K, "Toxicity of Lipid Peroxides in Processed Foods" in *Biochemical Reviews, Golden Jubilee Volume L*, Cama HR, et al, eds. (The Society of Biological Chemists, India, 1980), pp. 42-6

53. Freeman BA, Crapo JD, *Lab Invest* 47(1982): 412-26

54. Sharma HM, Alexander CN, *Research Review on Maharishi Ayur-Veda: A Comprehensive System of Natural Medicine* (Unpublished)

55. Ibid; Dybing E, et al, *Mol Pharmacol* 12(1976): 911-20; Levine, *Antioxidant* (see note 30), p. 241-2

56. Levine, *Antioxidant* (see note 30), p. 22

57. Southorn, *Mayo* (see note 3)

58. Levine, *Antioxidant* (see note 30), p. 19

59. Ibid, p. 285

60. Ibid, p. 287

CHAPTER THREE

Free Radicals, Aging, and Disease

To a practicing medical doctor, the symptoms of most diseases are well known. A disease-specific set of symptoms is sometimes called the *clinical presentation* of a disease—the way the illness appears when the patient comes to the clinic. Such clinical presentations are usually familiar, and only rarely are competent doctors unsure what disease they are facing.

When it comes to the cellular and subcellular events that give rise to a particular disease, however, the relevant facts have often been more obscure. The symptoms are obvious, but the cause is often unknown. For this reason, much of modern medicine has been devoted simply to the treatment of symptoms.

This is one reason why the free radical paradigm has been such a breakthrough in the field of medicine. By highlighting mechanisms of molecular damage, this new paradigm has provided insight into the initiation and progression of a wide range of diseases that had otherwise resisted clear understanding. Moreover, as we have seen, the understanding of free radical damage has provided a *single* explanation for diseases that, on clinical presentation, appear totally unrelated.

A decade ago it might have seemed absurd to argue that cataracts, rheumatoid arthritis, and strokes all have one basic source of damage in common, or that the etiology of cancer, heart disease, and dandruff share a common mechanism. But now the evidence for this unified understanding is compelling. For most of aging and disease, free radicals form the common link in the causal chain.

In fact, it now appears that the clinical presentation of different diseases may be due not to different causal mechanisms, but to variations in the protection provided by the body's antioxidant defenses. In a hurricane, the weakest link in a house will go—whether doors or windows or an insecure roof. Under oxidative stress, the weakest link in the body will give way. If free radical defenses are weak in the lungs, then oxidative stress may result in emphysema. If defenses are weak in the intestinal tract, then ulcerative colitis, Crohn's disease, or other inflammatory diseases of the digestive tract may appear. If defenses are weak in immune system cells, then the body will have less ability to fight infectious diseases. According to this view, doctors should look not so much for the cause of a disease as for a weakness in the body's defense systems.

To understand this new medical viewpoint, it is necessary to understand the specific mechanisms by which free radicals generate both disease and aging. And this understanding, in turn, begins with the mechanisms by which free radicals damage specific molecules in the cell. From the congestion of a cold to the terrors of cancer, the underlying reality is a war among the molecules.

DAMAGE TO PROTEINS

Cellular proteins are one of the primary free radical targets. Proteins make up a large portion of the structure of a cell, including the semi-rigid network of fibrils known as the cytoskeleton and a similar network within the nucleus known as the nuclear matrix. Muscles are protein, enzymes are protein, and most hormones and neurochemicals are protein, or largely protein. And all of this protein can be disfigured by free radicals. The precise molecular shapes of the proteins can be altered—or, in the biochemists' term, *denatured*—destroying their functionality.

The free radical attackers may hit at a particularly weak link in a protein, for example, and break the molecule in two. Or they may bite down on an electron and hold on permanently. This process, known as alkylation, creates an abnormal molecular shape. They may also take a bite and carry it away, leaving behind lesions in the attacked molecule. Such an electron robbery is like pulling out one card in a house of cards. The whole structure suddenly changes. The loss of a single electron from a single atom in a molecule can result in a chain reaction of adjustments that alters the molecular shape completely—destroying that molecule's biological usefulness. Finally, a species of two-fisted free radicals known as aldehydes can take hold of two molecules and link them together. This cross-linking creates stiff, inert piles of useless protein— producing the stiffening of ligaments and tendons that comes with aging.

Free radical damage is particularly destructive if it hits proteins known as *enzymes*—molecular machines that do useful work. Some enzymes manufacture large, complex molecules for use in the cell. Others take molecules apart, breaking them down into their raw materials to be recycled. If enzymes are damaged, that can cripple the cell's ability to function and keep its house in order.

DAMAGE TO DNA

The DNA molecule, being particularly delicate and complex, is especially vulnerable to free radical attack. At the core of the cell, the precisely coded strands of DNA are ordinarily sprawled out in a thread-like mass, like a ball of yarn after a kitten has had its way. Though it coils tightly when the cell divides, the DNA spreads itself out for everyday cell operations. It must be open and available so its coded information is accessible and ready for use. But this openness, coupled with the subtlety and precision of the DNA code, means that DNA molecules are an easy free radical target. A brief recounting of the DNA's coding system, and its mechanism for translating code into molecules, will reveal both the ingeniousness of cell operation and the dangers posed by free radical attack.[1]

The DNA code: The DNA code is carried by four molecules known as nucleotide bases—adenine, guanine, thymine, and cytosine. With the four molecules represented by the letters A, G, T, and C, each three-letter combination can be seen as a "word" or *codon;* this word corresponds to a particular amino acid available in the cell. Any particular sequence of three-letter words can be seen as a "sentence" or gene in the DNA which corresponds to a particular *sequence* of amino acids. When amino acids are joined together in the correct sequence, they form a specific protein. This means that each *gene* in the DNA (a particular sequence of three-letter codons) is a code for the amino acid sequence in a particular protein. DNA results in protein construction.

In the DNA coding mechanism, moreover, the code molecules themselves physically match up two by two. Adenine interlocks with thymine, and guanine with cytosine. DNA is actually a double strand, with every A in one strand matched by a T in the other, and every G with a C. The two strands are, in molecular metaphor, mirror images.

Making molecules: This code is used in a multi-step process. First, a particular string of codons in the DNA (a gene) gets copied off as messenger RNA (*ribonucleic acid*). The two DNA strands temporarily separate, exposing the proper sequence of codons. On this template, from atoms and molecular bits floating free in the nucleus, the mirror-image messenger RNA is formed. This messenger RNA has all the knowledge needed to produce a particular protein.

For every codon on this messenger RNA, there is yet another nucleic acid—transfer RNA. Each transfer RNA has a three-letter "identification card" that fits perfectly with its particular three-letter codon on the messenger RNA. The role of transfer RNA is to take hold of a specific amino acid, bring it to the messenger RNA, and lock it in sequence. Each transfer RNA will only take hold of one type of amino acid, and each fits only one codon on the messenger RNA. Thus, the amino acids are put together in the precise sequence dictated by the messenger RNA (and thus by the original gene in the DNA). The resulting string of amino acids is the correct protein.

Free radical attack: The entire mechanism, from DNA to the final components of the cell, is gloriously clever and efficient. But simply to recount this sequence is also to catalog a series of free radical targets. Working from the outside in, free radicals can attack completed components of the cell, disrupting cell operation; they can attack messenger and transfer RNA, disrupting the manufacturing process; and most dangerously, they can attack the DNA itself, altering the intelligence at the basis of all cell activities.

If the DNA itself is nicked—to use a geneticist's term for injury—then a gene can malfunction. If the sequence of A, T, G, and C is changed by translocations or deletions, the gene would then code for one or more incorrect amino acids.[2] A protein would be built with an incorrect sequence. Depending on the gene and protein involved, this could be a minor problem or it could be catastrophic. Just as likely, a damaged gene may cease to function altogether. One cell operation may simply cease to exist.

Free radicals can also damage both strands simultaneously, or break the polymer backbone of the double strand.[3] In addition, the entire DNA is surrounded by an enveloping cloud of proteins. These proteins are thought to move the DNA—as it positions itself to have a gene copied by RNA, for instance—and to provide pathways for the transportation of molecules within the nucleus.[4] These surrounding proteins can be cross-linked by free radicals, immobilizing them and restricting DNA function.[5]

DAMAGE TO CELL MEMBRANES

Free radical attack on cell membranes can be especially damaging. Attack on a single membrane molecule touches off a destructive chain reaction. The damage spreads down the membrane, and eventually results in a class of free radicals that move out to attack every vulnerable molecule in the cell.

Structure of cell membranes: Cell membranes are made up of long fatty molecules known as phospholipids. These membrane lipids are arranged in a double layer, with lipid tails in and phosphate heads out—like a double line of soldiers lying face down on the ground with feet together and heads apart. The phosphate head of each membrane lipid is attracted to water molecules. The heads of the outer layer thus face outward, into the water that surrounds each cell. The heads of the inner layer face inward, into the water within the cell. The long lipid tails of both layers, with no attraction to water, stick together in the middle of this membrane bilayer.

The cell's work surfaces: We have already seen that membranes can act as work surfaces, with enzymes embedded in the lipid bilayer. This is true not only in the mitochondria and the endoplasmic reticulum within the cell, but also in the outer cell membrane. This membrane is studded with protein complexes that have vital roles to play.

Some, for instance, are receptors, with specially shaped "hooks" sticking outside the cell into the intercellular spaces. When a molecule floats by that precisely matches the receptor, it hooks up temporarily with the receptor site. This, in turn, triggers a succession of changes in the receptor molecule and, eventually, within the cell. For example, if an epinephrine molecule is so received, the resulting changes within the cell lead to a decrease in normal housekeeping functions and an increase in energy production. If emergency chemotactic chemicals released by damaged cells begin to be picked up by receptors on immune system cells, those cells start moving toward higher concentrations of the emergency chemical. Receptors help cells talk with other cells—both nearby and throughout the body—and help to keep all cells everywhere in tune with each other.

Other protein complexes in the cell membrane act as pumps and transport mechanisms, ferrying molecules into and out of the cell. An important example is the sodium/potassium pump. This single system consumes up to 30% of the cell's energy supply. Its only function is to pump three positively charged sodium ions out of the cell for every two positively charged potassium ions it brings in. This may seem a trivial task to consume so much energy, but the result is that the fluid within the cell has a negative charge in comparison to the fluid outside the cell. This *ionic gradient* is vital to cell operation. The negative charge attracts the positive sodium ions back into the cell, and when they come they bring with them glucose molecules (fuel for the mitochondrial energy plants) and amino acids (the building blocks for all proteins). Without the sodium/potassium pump, the cell could not import its vital raw materials.

Free radical attack: When the cell membrane begins to unravel in a chain reaction caused by free radical attack, all these mechanisms are at risk. The damage starts at a kink in the long lipid chain that makes up the tail of each membrane lipid molecule. This kink is the weak link in the molecule. Where the chain suddenly bends, two carbon atoms are sharing four electrons, instead of the usual two. This is known as a *double bond*. It may sound stronger than a single bond but, as with much else in the sub-atomic, quantum mechanical world, appearances are deceiving. In fact, the electrons in this bond are not held as tightly as those elsewhere in the chain. In an instant, one of these electrons can be stolen, triggering a cascade of disastrous consequences.

Once the lipid has lost an electron, it is left with an unpaired electron. It becomes a free radical. Instantly, it readjusts its shape to fit the new situation, becoming forever ruined as a membrane component. It then takes up a complete oxygen molecule, but still retains an unpaired electron; biochemists call it a *lipid peroxy radical* at this phase—and it is an accident waiting to happen.

As heat energy bounces the molecules around, this radicalized lipid soon faces the vulnerable electron at the kink in its neighbor. It snatches that electron (along with its proton), and creates a new free radical.[6] Like a contagious disease, the unpaired electron status has been passed on.

Destructive chain reaction: At this stage, the damage elaborates in two directions. First, the progressive radicalization of lipid molecules proceeds down the cell membrane in a chain reaction. This can quickly compromise membrane function.[7] The membrane first becomes stiff and loses fluidity. Finally it breaks down altogether, leaking fluid and upsetting the ionic gradient in the cell.[8] The spreading radicalization can also attack protein complexes embedded in the cell membrane. As the free radical chain reaction spreads like a prairie fire, it destroys receptors, transport pumps, electron transport chains, and other critical mechanisms in its path.

In addition, each lipid that has been attacked and altered undergoes further deterioration of its own. Once the crippled molecule manages to steal an electron and proton from a neighboring lipid, it settles down for a while as relatively unreactive *lipid peroxide*. High levels of lipid peroxide circulating in the bloodstream are thus a good indication of ongoing free radical damage in the body.[9] Eventually, however, lipid peroxide deteriorates in one of two ways. First, it can break down into an aldehyde—the double-barreled molecule that has a free radical complex on each end. This aldehyde loses all connection with the membrane and floats freely anywhere in the cell, even into the nucleus. Its double free radical nature allows it to cross-link proteins and DNA, and destroy the function of enzymes by attaching stray bits of lipid to their structure.[10]

Lipid peroxide's other breakdown path is no more encouraging. In this sequence, it interacts with iron or copper to produce *two* free radicals—the alkoxy radical plus the hydroxy radical. The potential for additional damage has been at least doubled.

Cell membrane damage is thus deceptively destructive. The original chain reaction around the membrane is relatively slow; we have seen that the lipid peroxy radical has a half-life of seven seconds before it attacks a neighboring lipid—a lifetime trillions of times longer than the hydroxy radical. Despite this measured pace, the inexorable chain reaction around the membrane, the damage to membrane proteins, and the eventual cell-wide destruction caused by the aldehyde molecule and the other lipid peroxide breakdown products combine to make lipid oxidation one of the worst types of free radical damage. A single original attack by an oxy radical can theoretically result in cell death if the chain reaction is not checked.

THE SOURCE OF DISEASE

All this free radical damage is based on a single mechanism. A single quantum mechanical situation—electron hunger caused by an unpaired electron in an outer orbital—causes free radicals to damage biological molecules in many different ways. Furthermore, these basic molecular mechanisms manifest their effects upward through the various layers of the body.

First they appear as trauma to individual cells. This cell damage, in turn, manifests as damage to tissues, then to organs, and finally to entire physiological systems. When seen from the level of the body as a whole, the result is a functionally infinite variety of symptoms. By working at the basic molecular level of life, free radicals take advantage of powerfully destructive leverage. In the rest of this chapter we will review some of the major diseases caused by free radicals, as well as the free radical contribution to the aging process.

HEART DISEASE AND STROKE

Cardiovascular disease is the number one killer in America. In fact, heart and blood vessel diseases kill nearly one million Americans every year, almost as many as cancer, accidents, pneumonia, influenza, and all other causes of death combined. Nearly one in two Americans die of cardiovascular disease—one every 34 seconds. The American Heart Association estimates that this human tragedy translates into a total cost of $108.9 billion dollars per year—counting medical services, the cost of medications, and lost productivity.[11]

The underlying cause of most of this illness and suffering is atherosclerosis—the thickening of blood vessel walls that leads to stiffness, brittleness, and narrowing of the passageway. Just as calcium build-up in a water pipe can progressively reduce the flow of water in a pipe, so atherosclerosis in arteries can progressively reduce the flow of blood.

In recent years, there has been a great deal of publicity associating atherosclerosis with high levels of cholesterol in the bloodstream. But recent studies indicate that total cholesterol levels are not the primary issue. Healthy cholesterol, in fact, is much needed by the body to produce hormones, bile acids, and cell membranes. Circulating cholesterol (which consists of fatty lipoprotein molecules) is much like oil in an engine, providing a source of needed lubrication.

In successive experiments, the true nature of the problem has been narrowed down, first to a type of cholesterol known as low density lipoprotein (LDL)—as opposed to high density lipoprotein (HDL)—and then to *damaged* LDL. Recent work has shown that atherosclerosis actually correlates with circulating LDL that has been attacked by oxygen or free radicals—known as LDL-ox.[12] This rancid cholesterol is itself a free radical. Denham Harman, the free radical pioneer, was the first researcher to suggest free radical damage to lipoproteins is the major cause of atherosclerosis.[13] A flood of recent research has proven him right and revealed many steps in the process.[14]

Free radicals and atherosclerosis: Atherosclerosis begins with damage to artery walls. Oxygen and free radicals attack the lipids in endothelial (artery-lining) cell membranes. The cell membranes decompose due to the chain reaction of free radical damage. This cell damage pushes the chemotactic emergency button; lipid peroxide molecules set off the reactions that produce attractor molecules (while also creating more free radicals). Neutrophils and macrophages follow their noses to the scene, and release more free radicals and digestive enzymes which seriously increase the damage to endothelial cells in the artery wall.[15]

Meanwhile, circulating LDL gets involved in the spreading disorder. It may have already been oxidized and arrive as a free radical, or the chain reacting membranes in the arterial wall may attack it and turn it into a free radical.[16] In either event, LDL-ox is no longer recognized by receptors and cannot perform its major function—the deposit of lipid into cells.[17] Instead, LDL-ox begins to accumulate among damaged cells in the arterial wall.[18]

The picture is further complicated when macrophages, in pursuit of their janitorial duties, start to engulf the damaged

LDL. Being perhaps too assiduous, the macrophages stuff themselves with globules of these rancid fats; under a microscope the lipid-laden macrophages have a foamy appearance (these are referred to as *foam cells*).[19] Giving in to inertia, the bloated macrophages settle in amongst damaged cells in the arterial lining. Thus begins the deposit of fatty streaks on the arterial walls—streaks made of LDL-ox stuffed inside macrophages—the first serious sign of atherosclerosis.[20]

As the damaged arterial walls thicken with deposits of rancid fat, blood platelets are caught up in the biological trash. Platelets are small cells that circulate in the blood. At the site of any injury, they tend to clump together to stop the flow of blood. However, if these platelets have too great a tendency to aggregate, clots may form that block the flow of blood through the vessels themselves. Their unwanted tendency to aggregate in damaged arteries is encouraged by another free radical mechanism. Prostacyclin is produced by blood vessels and inhibits platelet aggregation. But free radical damage, principally by the hydroxy radical and radicalized lipids, inactivates prostacyclin—leaving platelets free to aggregate rapidly. In an area where, ideally, platelet aggregation could be minimized, the self-stimulating free radical activity instead makes it more likely.[21]

Blocked arteries: Arteries do not have to be totally blocked for major health problems to ensue. In the first place, all blood vessels are subject to *vasospasm* which constricts the flow of blood. Vasospasm has many causes, including stress and the ingestion of fatty foods. Under conditions of vasospasm, even lightly congested blood vessels can become nearly impassable, and seriously clogged vessels can be blocked altogether.

In the second place, when a blood vessel is partially blocked, this can cause *hypoxia* (reduced oxygen) in cells. During hypoxia, free radical damage in cells is very high. One cause is the mitochondrial electron transport chain. Reduced oxygen levels disrupt the smooth flow of the mitochondria's energy-creating chain. The oxygen levels are insufficient to keep pulling electrons off the bottom of the chain as quickly as necessary, so the chain backs up. Loose electrons pile up, especially at the head of the chain. Though oxygen is low, it is still available to interact with the loose electrons that have nowhere to go. Superoxide is created in abundance, leading soon to all other oxy radicals and ROS.[22]

Hypoxia also puts an important enzyme system through a Dr. Jekyll-Mr. Hyde transition. As part of the body's constant recycling process, xanthine dehydrogenase is responsible for breaking down purine bases (two of the code nucleotides in DNA are purine bases). When oxygen is low, however, xanthine dehydrogenase changes to xanthine oxidase.[23] Xanthine oxidase generates one superoxide molecule every time it breaks apart one purine molecule. Xanthine is everywhere in the cell, with especially high levels in the cell nucleus where it is needed to break down purines being recycled in the DNA. Once it has undergone its Mr. Hyde conversion, the damage caused by this free radical factory can be extremely serious.

When a blood vessel is totally blocked, the cell's oxygen supply is cut off completely. Available oxygen is soon used up. Like a computer that puts itself into the "sleep" mode to preserve battery power, the cell shuts down most basic operations and shifts over to the inefficient use of glycolysis to create a trickle of energy. Brain cells and a few other cell types cannot withstand this situation for more than a few minutes, but many cells can survive hours in this idling mode.

Reperfusion injury: When vasospasm hits a well-clogged artery leading to the heart, a heart attack can result. After a period of total lack of oxygen, the vasospasm may let up, allowing at least small amounts of blood to pass through. Then, when doctors administer streptokinase or other clot-dissolving drugs, the artery may suddenly open up wider. As mentioned in Chapter One, when blood returns to a formerly blood-starved area, either as a result of reduced vasospasm or clot-clearing chemicals, the paradoxical result is a sudden burst of extremely destructive free radical damage known as *reperfusion injury*.[24] Reperfusion injury causes serious damage to cell membranes, proteins, and DNA in the ventricles of the heart.[25] A study of 50 heart attack victims who received streptokinase showed that in 42 of them levels of lipid peroxide in the blood quickly rose—indicating a sudden increase in free radical damage.[26]

One reason for this is that during a period of complete oxygen starvation, levels of superoxide dismutase (SOD) in the cell go down. SOD's purpose is to defuse the free radical superoxide. If oxygen disappears, the superoxide radical also diminishes, and the DNA loses its signal to keep creating SOD. The SOD level drops dangerously. When oxygen suddenly returns to the cell and superoxide is suddenly created in large numbers at every electron transport chain, and by the xanthine oxidase enzyme, no SOD is there to stop it.

Although oxygen starvation and the ensuing reperfusion injury is dramatically noticeable in the heart, this type of injury can actually occur in many places in the body. It has been reported in the intestinal tract,[27] the kidney, and the central nervous system.[28]

Stroke: When blood vessels are narrowed and blood flow is restricted, brain cells are more seriously at risk than most other cells in the body. Brain cells have a low tolerance for hypoxia; cell death can occur quickly. If the clogged blood vessel combines with vasospasm to produce a total stoppage of blood, the brain cells can last only a matter of minutes. When atherosclerosis causes such trauma in the brain, the result is called a stroke. The American Heart Association estimates that half of all people hospitalized for acute neurological disease are victims of stroke.[29]

Since stroke is associated with lack of oxygen, excess free radicals can rapidly make the situation worse. One study has shown that those stroke victims whose levels of lipid peroxide in the bloodstream begin to fall in the days after the original attack have a good chance of survival. If the level of lipid peroxide continues to rise, survival is much less likely.[30] Increasing free radical activity indicates (and perhaps causes) continuing damage.

Cardiovascular summation: The mechanisms behind cardiovascular disease, America's number one killer, have thus been laid out in detail by a myriad of studies. Stripped to the essence, free radicals are central actors in the development of cardiovascular disease. They damage the blood vessel linings and LDL, attract white blood cells which increase the damage, cause the creation of foam cells full of LDL-ox, and encourage blood clotting. Once atherosclerosis has helped block an artery, the free radicals created by low-oxygen conditions within cells cause even more damage. If free radicals can be controlled, it should dramatically slow both the occurrence of, and the damage caused by, heart attacks, strokes, and other types of cardiovascular disease.

FREE RADICALS AND CANCER

Though cardiovascular disease affects more people than other diseases, cancer may be the more terrifying illness. Heart attack and stroke usually occur suddenly, without warning, and can be instantly fatal. Cancer, in comparison, is ordinarily slow and progressive. It is also peculiarly unsettling to many—a revolt of the body's cells against itself.

We have seen that the free radical mechanisms for creating cardiovascular disease are multi-layered and complex. The role free radicals play in the causation of cancer is much simpler. Free radicals attack the DNA. Cancer results.[31]

One of America's leading free radical researchers, Dr. Bruce Ames of the National Institute for Environmental Health Sciences at the University of California (Berkeley), estimates that the DNA in every cell in the human body is attacked by free radicals 10,000 times a day.[32] The risk therefore appears very large, yet cancer is, in comparison, quite rare. In fact, the important question seems to be not how cancer is caused, but why everyone doesn't fall ill with cancer immediately.

There are many reasons. First, the DNA repair mechanisms are extremely efficient—demonstrating a repair rate approaching 100% in healthy human beings. In the desperate battle to preserve its intelligence, the DNA has one strong advantage—its double-strand, positive-negative structure. If free radicals damage or release some of the code-carrying nucleotide molecules on one strand, DNA repair enzymes can use the second strand as a guide to repair the first. By matching A's to T's and G's to C's, the enzymes can reconstruct the damaged strand precisely. At least 50 enzymes are involved in such repair processes—and their efficiency is impressive. DNA repair in human beings is ordinarily close to perfect.[33]

Second, not every unrepaired attack on DNA results in cancer. Many nicks may have no noticeable effect at all, since large stretches of DNA have no purpose yet discovered. Others may cause an alteration or cessation of particular cell functions, without otherwise damaging the cell (we will return to this later). If the DNA damage is serious enough, on the other hand, the cell simply dies. It is only a particular type of damage that results in cancer.

The genetic fusebox: All cells in the body have the same set of genes coded in their DNA. Geneticists estimate that there are between 50,000 and 100,000 genes in every human cell. These genes are like a fusebox, however. In any given cell, relatively few of these genes are "switched on" (if a particular gene is "on," geneticists say it is *expressed*; if "off," it is *repressed*). A cell in the liver expresses only those genes that cause it to function as a liver cell. The same is true of specialized cells in, for example, the lung, stomach lining, or thigh muscle. Cells that are specialized in this way are said to be *dif-*

ferentiated. They are using those genes, and only those genes, that allow them to do their allotted tasks. Only those strips of messenger RNA are copied off the DNA that create the proteins needed by this particular type of cell.

When the DNA is damaged in such a way as to cause cancer, the cell usually loses its differentiated status. It is no longer a liver cell or a lung cell. The genes that lead to differentiation are switched off—either damaged or repressed—and the cell tends to the generic, capable of energy production and basic maintenance, but incapable of the particular tasks it was originally intended to perform. In most types of cancer, this undifferentiated cell also begins to reproduce much more rapidly. Though geneticists are not yet sure what type of genetic damage causes these traits, the result is dismaying—a strain of cells loose in the body that does no useful work and seems interested only in its own proliferation.

Even then, a strong immune system can stop much cancer before it gets out of control. Macrophages and other phagocytes recognize most cancer cells and digest them as if they were invaders. The immune system not only fights infection. It is also the last line of defense against cancer.

Free radicals in the initiation phase: Cancer has a two-phase growth process.[34] First is the initiation phase, in which apparently irreversible damage occurs to the DNA in one or more cells of a cell population. Second is the promotion phase, in which the damaged DNA is expressed through rapid reproduction of the new cell type. Free radicals are active in both of these phases.[35]

The initiation phase is often caused by chronic inflammation, a fact that has been known for many years but has only recently been explained. In chronic inflammation, white blood cells are constantly releasing showers of free radicals. The neutrophils and macrophages spew superoxide and hydrogen peroxide in all directions, and both can enter nearby cells and travel to the cell nucleus to damage genetic material. Hydroxy radicals and hypochlorous acid released in intercellular spaces have the same effect indirectly. They attack cell membranes externally—giving rise to a chain reaction of radicalized lipids and the eventual production of aldehydes that can travel inward to the nucleus and cross-link DNA and its surrounding proteins.[36]

Free radicals can be caught in the act of creating cancer by using *electron spin resonance* (ESR) spectrometers. The unbalanced electron spin caused by the unpaired electrons in free radicals shows up in these tests. Organs with excessive free radical activity appear as hot spots. In experiments in Russia, animals fed a carcinogenic diet showed an increase of free radicals in the liver, as measured by ESR. The levels increased for four months, after which cancer began in the liver.[37]

Two studies in America have also indicated the role of free radicals in the initiation of cancer. These studies found that people who live in areas with low soil levels of selenium, an important substance for anti-oxidant defense in the body (see Chapter Four), have a much higher incidence of cancer. The implication is that eating food and drinking water from soil that is rich in anti-oxidants may stop the damage caused by oxy radicals and ROS.[38] A Finnish study of 12,000 people over a four-year period provided confirmation. The study found that those people with the lowest levels of anti-oxidants in the bloodstream (vitamins A and E and selenium) were eleven times more likely to get cancer.[39]

The case against free radicals is also made by many anti-cancer drugs. Drugs such as adriamycin and bleomycin[40] work by releasing a cascade of free radicals in the nucleus of cancer cells.[41] One end of the molecule attaches firmly to the DNA within the cancer cell, while the other end takes on iron and uses it for a cycling reaction that mass produces hydroxy radicals and other damaging oxy species.[42]

Promotion phase: There is also evidence that cancer cells deliberately generate free radicals and ROS to speed their *metastasis*—their breakout from a local area. Cells isolated in the laboratory from various types of tumors have recently been shown to produce copious flows of hydrogen peroxide.[43] There is indirect evidence that cancerous cells still living in the body also produce free radicals and ROS; aggressive tumor cell populations increase their production of anti-oxidants—indicating a need to protect themselves against self-generated free radical levels.[44]

An increase of free radicals could break down the barriers that hem cancer cells in. In most areas of the body, cells and tissues are held together by collagen—a fibrous material made of protein. The University of California's Bruce Ames theorizes that free radicals and ROS could activate latent *collagenases*—enzymes that break down collagen. As these enzymes dissolved the collagen glue, local cells and tissues would separate. Cancer cells could escape and move easily to other areas of the body.[45]

Dr. Ames further indicates that, by deliberately creating free radicals and ROS, cancer cells can turn themselves into mutagen specialists—cells with a higher mutation rate. By attacking their own DNA, they can theoretically worsen their cancerous nature.[46]

OTHER DEGENERATIVE DISEASE

Extensive research has pointed the finger at free radicals as the cause of many other diseases—including every significant degenerative disease. The most important will be discussed here briefly, followed by a detailed free radical theory of the generalized aging process.

Rheumatoid arthritis. The body's joints have an organic version of a Teflon coating—synovial membranes that act as surface bearings. The joints are also filled with synovial fluid, which acts like grease in a hinge, and they have cartilage and collagen to act as shock absorbers. In arthritis, free radicals tear up all these mechanisms for smooth and painless functioning of the joints.

All arthritis is characterized by constant inflammation. Inflammation creates a constant flood of free radicals and ROS. The result is serious damage in the joints.[47] For example, superoxide degrades hyaluronic acid, a major component of the synovial fluid,[48] and it may do so by giving rise to the hydroxy radical.[49] The free radical attack also breaks down collagen in cartilage and connective tissue,[50] and damages endothelial cells lining the blood vessels of the joints.[51] Once this damage starts, moreover, if the free radical levels exceed local anti-oxidant defenses, the inflammatory response feeds on itself in a vicious cycle—and damage to the joint continues.

Free radicals generated by neutrophils have also been implicated as a cause of systemic lupus erythematosus, a generalized disorder of collagen-based connective tissue,[52] as well as inflammatory diseases of the digestive tract such as Crohn's disease and ulcerative colitis.[53]

Emphysema. Emphysema creates a loss of elasticity in lung tissue due to *fibrosis*, the stiffening and wrinkling caused by cross-linking of proteins. These damaged areas of the lung lose their ability to take in oxygen and release carbon dioxide and other gases. Emphysema has been related to free radical attack,[54] and the advance of emphysema is positively correlated with increases in lipid peroxide—the precursor of the cross-linking aldehyde.[55]

We have seen that certain types of chemicals in air pollution, especially ozone and nitrogen dioxide, arrive in the lungs as free radicals. Tobacco smoke also contains free radicals. In addition, the minute particulate matter in tobacco smoke lodges in the lungs where neutrophils and macrophages engulf it, spilling oxy radicals, ROS, and digestive enzymes in the process.[56] As is typical in the inflammatory reaction, free radicals break down the chemical meant to inhibit the digestive enzymes, and these enzymes cause much of the lung damage in emphysema.[57]

The lung damage precipitated by asbestos follows a similar pathway. The tiny asbestos particles attract white blood cells, leading to excessive oxy radical and ROS production. If a person continues to breathe asbestos, the reaction continues, leading to loss of lung function and often to cancer.[58]

Osteoporosis. Ninety-nine percent of the calcium in the body is ordinarily contained in bones and teeth. The one per cent circulating in the blood, however, has many significant functions in the body. Calcium helps regulate heartbeat, nervous system function, muscle control, enzyme systems, and hormone secretions, and helps cells to cohere and blood to coagulate. If the body does not have enough circulating calcium for these functions, it leaches it from the bones. This process can eventually lead to osteoporosis and frequent bone fractures. Research by Dr. Gregory Mudy at the University of Texas Health Center in San Antonio has shown that free radicals are involved in excessive leaching of bone calcium. When Dr. Mudy artificially stimulated free radical creation in bone tissue, bone loss increased. When he added SOD to scavenge superoxide, bone loss stopped. Keeping anti-oxidants high and oxidative stress low can apparently help to protect the body's bone structure.[59]

Diabetes. When beta cells in the pancreas fail to secrete enough insulin, the body loses its ability to metabolize carbohydrates and to reduce glucose levels in the bloodstream. Researchers believe that some people have weak free radical defenses in these beta cells, and that free radical damage to DNA in beta cells, resulting in dysfunction or cell death, helps cause maturity-onset diabetes. It is known, for example, that many chemicals—including alloxan, paraquat, and certain chemotherapeutic agents[60]—can stimulate excessive production of oxy radicals in the nuclei of beta cells. It is also recognized that higher levels of circulating lipid peroxide correlate with worse symptoms of diabetes[61]—indicating that free radicals are at work. Also, as we will see in the next chapter, anti-oxidants have been shown to ease the symptoms of diabetes.

Cataracts. Ultraviolet radiation in sunlight causes free radical activity which damages the eye's lens. Cataracts are especially prevalent in Tibet, for example, where thin air and a relatively treeless plateau expose the eye to greater ultraviolet radiation.[62] High levels of circulating lipid peroxide correlate with increased incidence of cataracts.[63]

Mental disorders. The brain is especially vulnerable to free radical damage.[64] Levels of vitamin C are 50 times higher in the brain than elsewhere in the body—possibly to help fight free radical damage.[65] Membranes in the brain are especially rich in the type of polyunsaturated fats that free radicals can attack. Neurons also have a high mitochondrial content, to sustain the vigorous activity needed for the brain's electrical functioning.[66] When these energy plants run, they create free radicals in abundance as inevitable toxic waste.

Since brain cells must live as long as the human body does, accumulated free radical damage to membranes, proteins, and DNA could degrade brain cell functioning over time—including the ability to secrete crucial neurotransmitter chemicals. We have seen that high levels of anti-oxidants administered to elderly gerbils resulted in a decrease in fractured proteins, an increase in secretion of neurotransmitters, and an improvement in learning ability.[67]

Free radicals have also been implicated in Parkinson's disease,[68] autism,[69] and schizophrenia.[70] One study of schizophrenics showed that 79% had high levels of circulating lipid peroxide and 86% had low levels of the anti-oxidant glutathione peroxidase in red blood cells.[71] Free radicals are a causative agent in many types of mental disorders.

A FREE RADICAL THEORY OF AGING

It has been said that people in our time fear aging more than death. In a culture that worships youth and vigorous health, the systematic collapse of the body and decline of the mind are particularly upsetting. These problems don't appear to bother the 97-year-old George Burns, who recently told an audience, "I'm glad to be here. I'm glad to be *anywhere.*" But the economic boom in exercise equipment, wrinkle creams, and cosmetic surgery clearly shows a widespread aversion to growing old.

A decade ago many gerontologists were still saying that aging has no apparent cause, and research evidence indicated that cells should continue to live forever. But at that time gerontologists were not focused at the molecular level. The free radical paradigm now allows a comprehensive theory of aging, a theory supported by considerable experimental data. We can now trace many of the aging mechanisms—if not all. More significantly, we can outline a program that may help dramatically slow the aging process.

To explore the details of this theory, it is best to start with a practical definition of aging. Rather than defining aging in terms of the mechanisms that cause it, we can focus on the observable results of aging. Aging causes (1) an increase in susceptibility to disease and (2) a decrease in physical functionality. Older people tend to get sick more. Older people have more trouble with hearing, eyesight, digestion, mental alertness, and other aspects of normal physical operation.

In one sense, therefore, this entire chapter has been about aging. The serious degenerative diseases ordinarily experienced during aging include cardiovascular disease, cancer, arthritis, diabetes, cataracts, osteoporosis, and mental degeneration. We have seen that free radicals are implicated in all these diseases. To the extent that aging means vulnerability to disease, free radicals are a major cause of aging.

Aging in cells: Free radicals also explain why youthful functioning slips away. We have seen that as cells age, oxidatively damaged proteins and other macromolecules are cross-linked into useless heaps which begin to pile up in the cell. These damaged molecules show up as increasing blobs of *lipofuscin*, or age pigment—yellowish or brownish spots that grow larger in the cells of older people, especially in the heart and brain.[72] Research suggests that increased age pigment correlates with decreased cell function—with a decrease, for instance, in neurotransmitters emitted by brain cells.[73]

This accumulation of age pigment in cells is directly proportional to the level of energy creation in the cell. The more electrons that roll down the mitochondrial electron transport chains, the more age pigment that builds up. The accumulation of such pigment is also inversely proportional to longevity. The more you have, the fewer years you survive.[74] Free radicals wear cells out.

From cells to the body as a whole: Looking cell by cell, it is difficult to determine how many are killed outright by free radical damage. Expired cells are broken up by the release of their own digestive enzymes and engulfed and cleared away by macrophages. Since the evidence is rapidly destroyed, the cause of death—even the fact of death—is hard to determine. It *can* be determined, on the other hand, that some older cells, even those clogged with lipofuscin, survive and maintain at least the normal housekeeping functions.[75]

Even if free radical damage is not lethal to all cells, it can be lethal to the organism as a whole. Though cells continue to exist, they can lose their usefulness. In addition, free radical injury in one area can lead to even greater injury in other areas. This damage builds up in tissues, organs, physiological systems, and the body as a whole.

Oxygen starvation: One key example is atherosclerosis. We have seen that free radical destructiveness produces narrowed, clotted blood vessels. But so far we have focused only on the damage atherosclerosis does to the heart and brain. Dr. Harry Demopoulos, a Professor of Pathology at New York University who has long been interested in free radical damage, reports that atherosclerosis can restrict blood flow to, and sap the vitality of, every organ in the body.

We all know that older people often become physically smaller, losing both bulk and height. Dr. Demopoulos points out that this shrinking process is dramatic in the major organs of the body. The brain shrinks from three pounds at maturity to two pounds in advanced age. The heart goes from 400 grams to 200. Similar shrinkage affects the liver, genitals, and even the skeletal bone structure.[76] It is also known that the most common cause of cell injury—from free radicals and other causes—is lack of oxygen.[77]

Dr. Demopoulos suggests that atherosclerosis occurring everywhere in the body systematically starves cells of oxygen and nutrients. If people experience chronically high levels of stress, the damage becomes worse. During stress, as we have seen, blood vessels leading to organs go into vasospasm; in badly clogged vessels this could lead to periods of total oxygen deprivation.

When the heart is deprived of oxygen, especially if initial damage is followed by reperfusion injury, the result can quickly be lethal. In other organs, serious damage can continue over a long period. Dr. Demopoulos theorizes that, as an ongoing and ever-increasing process, free radical-induced oxygen starvation of cells leads to the systematic wasting away of tissues and organs. The body is slowly strangled by atherosclerosis.

Loss of cell memory: Dr. Richard Cutler of the National Institute for Aging (NIA) emphasizes a related pathway for cumulative damage to the organism as a whole. He points out that the complex human physiology, made of many different types of cells, stems originally from a single, undifferentiated cell. Somehow, as that single cell begins to rapidly divide and multiply, cells begin to differentiate. The first cells are all the same, but later cells specialize as liver cells, brain cells, muscle cells, etc. The process of growth and development involves the ability of cells in specific areas to specialize—to differentiate. Increasing cell differentiation is thus a hallmark of the creation and maturation of the body.

Dr. Cutler suggests that the reverse process, which he calls *dysdifferentiation*—the progressive reversion of cells toward non-specific status—may be one major characteristic of aging and decay. Cells may forget their specialized roles and, in whole or in part, degenerate toward generic cells (with or, more commonly, without the uncontrolled reproduction that is characteristic of cancer cells).[78] "Aging may be a process of losing ourselves," Dr. Cutler says. "As genes turn on or off incorrectly, each cell loses its ability to maintain its proper differentiation."[79]

Research has shown that the number of completely dysdifferentiated cells increases with the age of the organism.[80] But major damage could occur even without complete reversion to generic status. If the cell drifts only slightly from its perfectly tuned status, it might, for example, lose its ability to respond to specific hormones or perform allotted tasks.

As mentioned above, the differentiated status of a cell depends on which genes are expressed and which are not. Dr. Cutler's work has shown that oxy radicals and ROS can damage the DNA and alter the differentiated state of a cell at extremely low concentrations, and that anti-oxidant substances protect the cell from this genetic alteration.[81] Thus, oxidative stress is a plausible cause of dysdifferentiation throughout the body. Excess free radicals can turn our cells into functionless neuters.

The aging multiplier: Unfortunately, such damage can be multiplied manyfold. The negative effects of both oxygen starvation and dysdifferentiation are greatest when they affect physiological systems closely tied to the overall aging process. The two most important systems of this type are (1) the neuroendocrine system regulated by the hypothalamus and (2) the immune system. When these systems deteriorate, they take the entire body with them.

Hormone starvation: Many of the body's hormones are necessary to maintain healthy, youthful functioning—including growth hormone, adrenocorticotropic hormone, thyroid-stimulating hormone and dehydroepiandrosterone sulfate (DHEA-S). Most of these hormones are secreted by the pituitary gland at the base of the brain. The pituitary, in turn, takes its biochemical orders from the hypothalamus, the brain's central regulating agency.[82]

Dr. Caleb Finch of the University of Southern California has shown that the hypothalamus in older animals releases smaller amounts of neurotransmitters necessary to stimulate pituitary activity.[83] As the pituitary then emits less of its hormonal messengers, other glands also slow, and the body as a whole is deprived of needed chemicals.

Dr. Cutler of the NIA suggests that progressive dysdifferentiation of cells in the hypothalamus and pituitary could account for this progressively diminishing output of neurotransmitters and hormones.[84] Such dysdifferentiation could be caused by direct free radical attack on the DNA of cells in the hypothalamus and pituitary. In addition, generalized atherosclerosis could accelerate this process. Because these cells are crucial to the operation of the entire body, only a small number damaged produce significant loss of physical function. When free radicals damage the hypothalamus and pituitary, aging accelerates exponentially.

Immune malfunction: Malfunction in the immune system can also speed the overall process of aging. Over the course of time, the immune system degrades in two ways. First, it progressively loses its ability to fight infectious disease. Second, and more treacherously, it begins to attack the body itself. The receptors in white blood cells malfunction and no longer do an accurate job of discriminating between the chemical markers of friend and foe. They aim their powerful free radical cascades at the body's own cells.

The influence of such age-related malfunction has been shown in experiments with laboratory mice. When white blood cells from aged mice were injected into very young mice, the younger mice displayed graying fur, liver and kidney disease, and shortened life span.[85]

What accounts for this degeneration of the immune system with age? One theory is that cells in this system could easily be subject to the same sort of dysdifferentiation seen in other parts of the body, where genes are incorrectly turned on or off. In the immune system cells, such dysdifferentiation could produce immune cells that attack the wrong enemy, or fail to attack at all.

In this case, moreover, researchers have identified a crucial sector of the genetic code. It is called the *major histocompatibility complex* (MHC) and it influences the immune system, free radical defenses, and, some evidence indicates, DNA repair.[86] Dr. Roy Walford, a researcher on aging at the University of California at Los Angeles, has shown that relative life span among different strains of mice is directly related to differences in the MHC.[87] Diseases of aging, including senile dementia, are more likely when people have a particular type of MHC.[88] Also, a disease we have already mentioned, systemic lupus erythematosus (lupus), generates many of the features of accelerated aging. Susceptibility to this disease is controlled in part by the MHC. The symptoms of lupus can be inhibited by the use of SOD for control of free radical generation.[89]

Dr. Walford cites such evidence when he suggests that because the MHC is so closely related to the immune system and free radical defenses, as well as aging, it might better be called the Life Support Complex. Dr. Walford explains that progressive free radical damage to the MHC (a particularly crippling example of dysdifferentiation), passed on and increasing from one cell generation to the next, could impair functioning of the immune system and reduce the body's anti-oxidant defenses.

Weakening of the anti-oxidant defenses would have negative effects everywhere in the body. Specifically:

1. It would weaken the immune system by reducing the protection immune cells need to keep their oxy radical weapons from damaging themselves.

2. It would reduce the protection enjoyed by the whole body against immune system excesses.

3. It would increase free radical attack on immune system DNA, producing mutations that would cause them to attack normal cells instead of invaders.

The systematic result would be loss of immune system functioning combined with generalized damage all over the body. Dysdifferentiation in the MHC could have drastic effects on the aging rate of the organism as a whole.

By killing cells outright, or weakening their ability to perform their assigned duties, free radicals thus speed the aging process. Damage can occur in any cell in the body, but when it hits crucial systems, the rate of aging becomes exponential. Though these mechanisms may not explain all of aging, the research indicates they have a major effect.

With this review of the free radical role in illness and aging, we have fulfilled the purpose of Part One. We have described the molecular environment of free radicals in human cells, the sources of free radicals, and the damage they render. We know now what the problem is. The question becomes what to do about it.

It is time to learn how to bring free radicals under control.

Notes

1. This chapter briefly reviews several of the most basic aspects of molecular structure and activities in the cell—information available in any basic textbook on the subject. For lay readers interested in further detail, I recommend books from the *Scientific American* series: Atkins PW, *Atoms, Electrons, and Change* (Scientific American Library, New York, 1991); Atkins PW, *Molecules* (Scientific American Library, New York, 1987); de Duve C, *A Guided Tour of the Living Cell, Volumes 1 & 2* (Scientific American Library, New York, 1984). For more substance, an excellent university textbook, well organized and clearly written, is: Alberts B, et al, *Molecular Biology of the Cell* (Garland Publishing, Inc., New York, 1983)

2. Fantone JC, Ward PA, *Current Concepts: Oxygen-Derived Radicals and Their Metabolites: Relationship to Tissue Injury* (The Upjohn Company, Kalamazoo, 1985), p. 36

3. Burger RM, et al, *Life Sci* 28(1981): 715-27; Lin PS, et al, *Cancer* 46(1980): 2360-4

4. Pienta KJ, Coffey DS, *Med Hypotheses* 34(1991): 88-95

5. Walford RL, *Maximum Life Span* (Avon, New York, 1983), p. 168

6. Diplock AT, *Am J Clin Nutr* 53(1991): 189S-93S; Niki E, et al, *Am J Clin Nutr* 53(1991): 201S-5S; Di Máscio P, et al, *Am J Clin Nutr* 53(1991): 194S-200S; Luc G, Fruchart J-C, *Am J Clin Nutr*, 53(1991): 206S-9S

7. Mead JF, "Free Radical Mechanisms of Lipid Damage and Consequences for Cellular Membranes" in *Free Radicals in Biology, Vol. 1*, Pryor WA, ed. (Academic Press, New York, 1976), pp. 51-68

8. Maridonneau I, et al, *J Biol Chem* 258(1983): 3107-13

9. Yagi K, "Assay for Serum Lipid Peroxide Level and its Clinical Significance" in *Lipid Peroxides in Biology and Medicine*, Yagi K, ed. (Academic Press, New York, 1982), pp. 223-42

10. Neilsen H, *Lipids* 16(1981): 215-222

11. *1992 Heart and Stroke Facts* (American Heart Association, 1991)

12. Levine SA, Kidd PM, *Antioxidant Adaptation: Its Role in Free Radical Pathology* (Biocurrents Division, Allergy Research Group, San Leandro, 1986), p. xi

13. Harman D, "The Free-Radical Theory of Aging" in *Free Radicals in Biology, Vol. 5*, Pryor WA, ed. (Academic Press, New York, 1982), pp. 255-75

14. Luc, *Am J Clin Nutr* (see note 6); Riemersma RA, et al, *Lancet* 337(1991): 1-5; Jialal I, et al, *Atherosclerosis* 82(1990): 185-91

15. Till GO, et al, *J Clin Invest* 69(1982): 1126-35; Johnson A, et al, *Am J Pathol* 114(1984): 410-7; Ward PA, et al, *J Clin Invest* 72(1983): 789-801; Perkowski SZ, et al, *Circ Res* 53(1983): 574-83; Till GO, et al, *J Trauma* 23(1983): 269-77

16. Southorn P, Powis G, *Mayo Clin Proc* 63(1988): 390-408

17. Hooper C, *J NIH Res* 1(1989): 101-6; Stringer M, et al, *Br Med J* 298(1989): 281-4

18. Morel DW, et al, *Arterioscl* 4(1984): 357-64; Steinbrecher UP, et al, *Proc Nat'l Acad Sci USA* 81(1984): 3883-7

19. Kita T, "Lipoprotein Metabolism in the WHHL Rabbit; An Animal Model for Familial Hypercholesterolemia" in *Atherosclerosis VII*, Fidge NH, Nestel PJ, eds. (Elsevier, Amsterdam, 1986), pp. 227-30; Yokode M, et al, in *Advances in Prostaglandin, Thromboxane and Leukotriene Research*, Samuelsson B, et al, eds. (Medical and Scientific Publishers, New York, 1987)

20. Brown MS, Goldstein JL, *Annu Rev Biochem* 52(1983): 223-61; Kita T, et al, *J Clin Invest* 77(1986): 1460-5; Steinberg D, *Arterioscl* 3(1983): 283-301; Goldstein JL, et al, *Proc Nat'l Acad Sci USA* 76(1979): 333-7; Brown MS, et al, *J Cell Biol* 82(1979): 597-613; Fogelman AM, et al, *Proc Nat'l Acad Sci USA* 77(1980): 2214-8

21. Stringer, *Br Med* (see note 17); Cotran RS, et al, eds., *Robbins Pathologic Basis of Disease* (W.B. Saunders Co., Philadelphia, 1989)

22. Niwa Y, Tsutsui D, *Saishinigaku* (Japan) 38(1983): 1450-8

23. McCord JM, Roy RS, *Can J Physiol Pharmacol* 60(1982): 1346-52

24. Burrell CJ, Blake DR, *Br Heart J* 61(1989): 4-8; Davies SW, "Free Radicals and Myocardial Disease–Studies in Patients" in *Free Radicals, Diseased States and Anti-Radical Interventions*, Rice-Evans C, ed. (Richelieu Press, London, 1989), pp. 97-115

25. Meerson FZ, et al, *Biull Eksp Biol Med* 92(1981): 281-3 (Russian, with English abstract); Davies SW, et al, *Lancet* 335(1990): 741-3

26. Guarnieri C, et al, *J Mol Cell Cardiol* 12(1980): 797-808

27. Grogaard B, et al, *Am J Physiol* 242(1982): G448-54

28. DeWall RA, et al, *Am Heart J* 82(1971): 362-70; Lefer AM, et al, *Circ Shock* 8(1981): 273-82; McCord, *Can* (see note 23); Fantone, *Current* (see note 2), p. 32

29. *1992 Heart* (see note 11)

30. Goto Y, "Lipid Peroxides as a Cause of Vascular Diseases" in *Lipid Peroxides in Biology and Medicine*, Yagi K, ed. (Academic Press, New York, 1982), pp. 295-303

31. Diplock, *Am J* (see note 6); Niki, *Am J* (see note 6); Di Mascio, *Am J* (see note 6); Luc, *Am J* (see note 6); Weisburger JH, *Am J Clin Nutr* 53(1991): 226S-37S

32. Ames BN, Shigenaga MK, "DNA Damage by Endogenous Oxidants and Mitogenesis As Causes of Aging and Cancer" in *Molecular Biology of Free Radical Scavenging Systems*, Scandalios JG, ed. (Cold Spring Harbor Laboratory Press, Plainview, 1992), pp. 1-21

33. Ibid

34. Southorn, *Mayo*, (see note 16)

35. Fischer S, et al, *Cancer Res* 48(1988): 3882-7; Floyd R, *FASEB* 4(1990): 2587-97

36. Weitzman SA, et al, *Science* 227(1985): 1231-3; Southorn, *Mayo*, (see note 16)

37. Emanuel NM, "Free Radicals During Appearance and Growth of Tumors" in *Free Radicals and Cancer*, Floyd RA, ed. (Marcel Dekker, Inc., New York, 1982), pp. 245-319; Shulyakovskaya TA, et al, *Dokl Akad Nauk, USSR* 210(1973): 221-3

38. Shamberger RJ, et al, *Arch Environ Health* 31(1976): 231-5; Schrauzer GN, et al, *Bioinorg Chem* 7(1977): 23-31

39. Salonen JT, et al, *Brit Med J* 290(1985): 417-20

40. Ishida R, Takahashi T, *Biochem Biophys Res Commun* 66(1975): 1432-8; Sugiura Y, Suzuki T, *J Biol Chem* 257(1982): 10544-6

41. Ferrans VJ, *Adv Exp Med Biol* 161(1983): 519-32; Von Hoff DD, et al, *Am J Med* 62(1977): 200-8; Lefrak EA, et al, *Cancer* 32(1973): 302-14

42. Burger, *Life* (see note 3); Lin, *Cancer* (see note 3)

43. Szatrowski TP, Nathan CF, *Cancer Res* 51(1991): 794-8

44. Borunov EV, et al, *Biull Eksp Biol Med* 107(1989): 467-9 (Russian, with English abstract)

45. Ames, *DNA* (see note 32)

46. Ibid

47. Cross CE, et al, *Ann Intern Med* 107(1987): 526-45

48. Greenwald RA, Moy WW, *Arthritis Rheum* 23(1980): 455-63

49. Halliwell B, "Free Radicals, Oxygen Toxicity, and Aging" in *Age Pigments*, Sohal RS, ed. (Elsevier—North Holland Biomedical Press, Amsterdam, 1981), pp. 1-62; Halliwell B, *Bull Europ Physiopath Resp* 17 (Supplement)(1981): 21-9

50. Greenwald RA, Moy WW, *Arthritis Rheum* 22(1979): 251-9

51. del Maestro RF, et al, "Free Radicals and Microvascular Permeability" in *Pathology of Oxygen*, Autor AP, ed. (Academic Press, New York, 1982), pp. 157-73; Fligiel SEG, et al, *Fed Proc* 43(1984): 954 (Abstract)

52. Niwa Y, et al, *Inflammation* 9(1985): 163-72

53. Niwa Y, Hanssen M, *Protection for Life: How to Boost Your Body's Defences Against Free Radicals and the Ageing Effects of Pollution and Modern Lifestyles* (Thorsons Publishers, Ltd., Wellingborough, 1989), p. 18

54. Cross, *Ann* (see note 47)

55. Oxygen Free Radicals and Tissue Damage (Ciba Foundation Symposium 65)(Excerpta Medica, Amsterdam, 1979)

56. Weiss SJ, LoBuglio AF, *Lab Invest* 47(1982): 5-18; Fantone JC, Ward PA, *Am J Pathol* 107(1982): 395-418

57. Southorn, *Mayo* (see note 16); Fantone, *Current* (see note 2), pp. 1-51

58. Roney PL, Holian A, *Toxicol Appl Pharmacol* 100(1989): 132-44

59. Hooper, *J NIH* (see note 17)

60. Farrington JA, et al, *Biochim Biophys Acta* 314(1973): 372-81; Pyatak PS, et al, *Res Commun Chem Pathol Pharmacol* 29(1980): 113-27; Fisher HK, et al, *Ann Intern Med* 75(1971): 731-6; Ishida, *Biochem* (see note 40); Sugiura, *J Biol* (see note 40); Ferrans, *Adv* (see note 41); Von Hoff, *Am* (see note 41); Lefrak, *Cancer* (see note 41)

61. Sato Y, et al, *Biochem Med* 21(1979): 104-7

62. Niwa, *Protection* (see note 53)

63. Yagi K, *Clin Chim Acta* 80(1977): 355-60

64. Seligman ML, et al, *Lipids* 12(1977): 945-50

65. Kronhausen E, et al, *Formula for Life* (William Morrow and Co., Inc., New York, 1989), p. 76

66. Demopoulos HB, et al, "Oxygen Free Radicals in Central Nervous System Ischemia and Trauma" in *Pathology of Oxygen*, Autor AP, ed. (Academic Press, New York, 1982), pp. 127-55

67. Carney JM, et al, *Proc Nat'l Acad Sci USA* 88(1991): 3633-6

68. Fahn S, *Am J Clin Nutr* 53(1991): 380S-2S

69. Levine, *Antioxidant* (see note 12), pp. 192-3

70. Hoffer A, *J Orthomol Psychiatry* 12(1983): 292-301

71. Pecora P, Shriftman MS, *A Study of Insulin, Fatty Acids and Other Metabolites in Psychiatric and Normal Control Populations* (Monroe Medical Research Laboratory, Monroe, 1983)

72. Taubald RD, et al, *Lipids* 10(1975): 383-90

73. Carney, *Proc* (see note 67)

74. Southorn, *Mayo*, (see note 16)

75. Cutler RG, "Longevity is Determined by Specific Genes: Testing the Hypothesis" in *Testing the Theories of Aging*, Adelman R, Roth G, eds. (CRC Press, Boca Raton, 1982), pp. 25-114; Cutler RG, "The Dysdifferentiative Hypothesis of Mammalian Aging and Longevity" in *The Aging Brain: Cellular and Molecular Mechanisms of Aging in the Nervous System*, Aging Vol. 20, Giacobini E, et al, eds. (Raven Press, New York, 1982), pp. 1-19; Cutler RG, "Dysdifferentiation and Aging" in *Molecular Biology of Aging: Gene Stability and Gene Expression*, Sohal RS, et al, eds. (Raven Press, New York, 1985), pp. 307-40

76. Kronhausen, *Formula* (see note 65), p. 223

77. Cotran, *Robbins* (see note 21), pp. 2-12

78. Cutler RG, *Am J Clin Nutr* 53(1991): 373S-9S

79. Richard G. Cutler, Biochemist, National Institute on Aging, personal communication (June 1992)

80. Cutler, *Am* (see note 78)

81. Ibid

82. Guyton AC, *Textbook of Medical Physiology, Eighth Edition* (W.B. Saunders Co., Philadelphia, 1991), pp. 819-30

83. Walford, *Maximum* (see note 5), p. 90

84. Cutler, (see note 79)

85. Walford, *Maximum* (see note 5), p.93

86. Smith GS, Walford RL, *Nature* 270(1977): 727-9; Williams RM, et al, "Genetics of Survival in Mice: Localization of Dominant Effects to Sub-regions of the Major Histocompatibility Complex" in *Immunological Aspects of Aging*, Segre D, Smith L, eds. (Dekker Publishing Company, New York, 1981): 247-66

87. Smith, *Nature* (see note 86)

88. Walford, *Maximum* (see note 5), p. 94

89. Emerit I, Michelson AM, *Proc Nat'l Acad Sci USA* 78(1981): 2537-40

PART TWO

Winning the Battle

CHAPTER FOUR

The Body's Defenses

In this section of the book, anti-oxidant defenses come to the rescue. There is no need to sit back passively while our molecules are destroyed. For those who would like to live longer, and live *younger* longer, thousands of studies on free radicals and free radical management now indicate there are effective steps to take—steps we will cover in the next three chapters.

First, we will review the body's own internal systems for defense against free radicals. Second, we will cover additional defense troops your body can import (vitamins and other nutrients) to tip the balance in its favor. Finally, we will analyze free radical prevention—the use of stress management to stop these molecular sharks before they get started. Taken together, these chapters contain a recipe for free radical control.

They also report the startling research that first interested me in the free radical field. Free radicals are one of the most recent discoveries of modern science—but research indicates they are controlled most effectively by an ancient system of natural health care. Comparative laboratory research and long-term insurance studies have shown that nutritional and stress management programs stemming from the traditional ayurvedic system of India clearly neutralize free radicals with unique effectiveness. In this section we will cover in detail this conjunction of modern science with ancient wisdom.

I am convinced that everyone should be aware of the scientific discoveries covered in the next three chapters. We now have the knowledge to transform our physical and mental health. But that doesn't mean that everyone should become his or her own medical expert. Nothing in this book is meant to replace the advice of a physician. If you are sick, go to a doctor. In the back of this book, you will find lists of organizations you can call to find medical doctors who are familiar with the free radical paradigm and natural prevention. It *is* possible to have the best of both worlds.

THE ENZYME ARMY

A strong anti-oxidant system is a bedrock necessity for oxygen-based life. Even unicellular organisms could never have made the Faustian bargain with oxygen had they not developed free radical defense. Every organism that lives with oxygen has systems for defusing the danger—but the level of efficiency varies widely. Mice aren't very good at stopping free radicals, for example. Every day they take ten times as many free radical hits on each DNA molecule as humans do.[1] They live only a few years. Human beings are relatively good at it. We live much longer.

The body has three lines of defense to combat free radicals once they have been generated:

1. The first line consists of enzyme systems—molecular machinery built by the body to specifications maintained in the DNA. These enzymes take free radicals apart, or blunt their sting.

2. The second line consists of a wide range of internally created biomolecules which quench the free radical thirst for electrons by giving up electrons of their own. These are known as extracellular free radical quenchers. Such molecules are sacrificial, donating an electron so crucial molecules in the cell might keep theirs.

3. The last line of defense is nutrients—molecules the body ingests ready-made. These supplemental reinforcements also work through the sacrificial mode.

Within the enzymatic line of defense, there are three major enzymes:

1. Superoxide dismutase, which focuses on the master free radical, superoxide.

2. Catalase, which specializes in hydrogen peroxide (strictly speaking, a reactive oxygen species or ROS, rather than a free radical).

3. Glutathione peroxidase, which can deal with both hydrogen peroxide and the lipid peroxides generated in cell membranes.

These enzymes are thousands of times more effective, molecule for molecule, than sacrificial biochemicals or nutrients.[2] As an example, when vitamin E gives up an electron to satisfy a ravenous free radical, it has done all it can on its own. It has become, in fact, a free radical itself, its lost electron leaving one unpaired behind (though its molecular conformation makes it relatively unreactive). Such oxidized vitamin E is stale and useless. It can return to the fray, but only if it can find a replacement electron.

Enzymes, on the other hand, do their work of altering free radicals and ROS without themselves being changed. They pull their prey in, disarm them, and let them go. Catalase, for example, pulls in hydrogen peroxide, H_2O_2. It snips off an oxygen, leaving the safe and stable water (H_2O), and marries the severed oxygen molecule to a second oxygen molecule, producing molecular oxygen.[3] Catalase is immediately ready to do its work again. Anti-oxidant enzymes may cause thousands of such molecular alterations before constant pounding by other molecules in the cell (due to heat motion) begins to break them down.

These enzyme defense forces have several admirable traits. First is their huge capacity for work. Second, the DNA keeps relatively high numbers of these enzymes in circulation at all times. They can react immediately to quench a free radical outbreak. Third, they are *inducible*—large numbers of them can be created rapidly by the DNA in response to a sudden increase in the free radical population.[4] On the other hand, these enzymes do have limitations. None of them can directly disarm the instantaneously destructive hydroxy radical, for example, and none of them deals with singlet oxygen.[5]

Further details on the anti-oxidant enzymes follow.

Superoxide dismutase (SOD). The discovery of SOD in animal cells was a major landmark in developing the free radical paradigm. Prior to this, the presence of free radicals in animal and human cells was questioned. But SOD has only one purpose: to stop the superoxide free radical. By scavenging this master free radical assiduously, SOD can stop its damage and, more significantly, head off reactions that result in formation of the much more reactive hydroxy radical.

SOD works by adding to superoxide, rather than breaking it up. Superoxide is molecular oxygen that has stolen an extra, unpaired electron ($O_2^{\bullet}$). SOD takes a firm grip on the superoxide molecule, attaches a proton to that extra electron, making it a hydrogen atom, then affixes a second hydrogen atom. The result is two hydrogens and two oxygens, H_2O_2, hydrogen peroxide.

This is a natural reaction which superoxide would undergo in any event, but SOD makes the reaction happen at ten million times its spontaneous rate.[6] The product of this reaction, hydrogen peroxide, is itself a reactive oxygen species (ROS) of intermediate reactivity. It can cause significant damage in sufficient quantities. SOD may not seem to be doing the best possible job, leaving an ROS in its wake. But SOD has back-up support, as we will see.[7]

Research has clearly shown that SOD defends the body valiantly. It guards against cancer, protects immune system cells, and guards the lungs. Because free radical damage can be so widespread, effective free radical defense can seem almost miraculous. The studies on SOD first made that obvious.

To begin with, higher levels of SOD correlate with reduced cancer.[8] By reducing levels of superoxide, SOD reduces creation of its hydroxy radical descendant—thus protecting DNA from hydroxy radical damage. In addition, adding SOD to a system including activated immune system cells, such as neutrophils and macrophages, reduces the mortality rate those immune cells suffer. By scavenging superoxide, SOD reduces free radical damage that phagocytes often do to themselves.[9]

DNA can react to increased free radical attacks by inducing increased levels of SOD.[10] In one experiment in Japan, 16 cigarette smokers were locked in a room playing cards for 18 hours. Their level of free radical activity increased dramatically. In 14 of the 16, SOD levels rose dramatically as well.[11]

SOD can also protect against excess oxygen. We have seen that breathable oxygen becomes lethal at high concentrations. As the percentage of oxygen in the air we breathe increases from 20%, which is normal in the atmosphere, toward 100%, serious damage begins to accumulate in the lungs. Free radical generation produces cross-linking of molecules and lack of flexibility in lung tissue.

In laboratory animals, tolerance for such high levels of oxygen is higher in young rats because they respond more quickly with higher levels of SOD.[12] SOD and catalase administered together can save animals even when they are breathing 100% oxygen.[13] The ability of SOD to suppress oxygen toxicity has also been indicated directly in lung tissue experiments.[14]

It has also been shown that people who respond to burns by producing high levels of SOD recover from their wounds more quickly. One reason is that SOD scavenges excess free radicals and slows lipid peroxidation damage to neighboring cells; this, in turn, reduces the level of emergency chemicals which damaged cells emit to attract more immune system cells.[15] SOD thus works to keep the inflammation reaction under control, reducing unnecessary damage.

In burn victims with low levels of SOD, healing is much slower.[16] If SOD levels are low, moreover, the scar tissue produced is lumpy. When SOD levels are high, burns heal smoothly.[17] As the body ages, however, its ability to induce SOD on demand appears to decline. Baseline levels don't drop much, but in an emergency SOD is not produced as rapidly. As a result, elderly burn victims show lower levels of SOD and slower healing.[18]

Catalase. In the history of free radical study, catalase was the second enzyme to get significant attention. It was once thought to be a major player in anti-oxidant defense for the cell as a whole. More recently, however, studies seem to indicate that catalase has only a peripheral role.[19]

Catalase breaks down hydrogen peroxide into water and oxygen. But catalase is only available within sub-cellular organelles known as peroxisomes. These microbodies have an extremely primitive system for oxidizing foodstuffs—a system which wastes all its energy creation as heat. This primitive oxidation, moreover, creates hydrogen peroxide as an integral by-product of the main reaction—thus requiring high concentrations of catalase simply to keep the peroxisomes functioning. Some researchers speculate that peroxisomes, like mitochondria, were once independent organisms, but earlier and less sophisticated on the evolutionary scale. In any event, catalase has its hands full breaking down hydrogen peroxide made within the peroxisome itself.[20]

It is likely that some hydrogen peroxide from elsewhere in the cell is also broken down by catalase after traveling to the peroxisomes. But this seems inherently inefficient—why would hydrogen peroxide meekly travel to peroxisomes without causing trouble before arriving? Research indicates that this process does not play a significant part in general anti-oxidant defenses. In the first place, although longer-lived organisms contain markedly higher concentrations of SOD and some other anti-oxidants, they do not contain higher concentrations of catalase.[21] This indicates that catalase does not have to be increased to provide better defense against free radicals. In the second place, organisms with hereditary acatalasemia (a total absence of catalase) have no impairment in their ability to deal with free radical attacks.[22] Catalase is like a slingshot on a modern battlefield; it doesn't hurt to have it, but it rarely does much good.

Glutathione peroxidase. The third anti-oxidant enzyme to gain major attention is part of an enzyme system which, in the view of many biochemists, is at least as important as SOD. All components of the glutathione system are at very high concentrations throughout every cell. This is especially true in the liver, where the body detoxifies poisonous molecules, often at the cost of producing free radicals and hydrogen peroxide.[23] Glutathione peroxidase is also highly inducible, like SOD, being generated rapidly when oxidative stress increases.[24]

Glutathione peroxidase performs two vital jobs. First, it dismantles hydrogen peroxide everywhere in the cell—thus finishing the business started by SOD.[25] Without this second step, SOD's transformation of superoxide into hydrogen peroxide would actually be dangerous. By the time SOD transformed half a given concentration of superoxide, for example, superoxide and hydrogen peroxide would coexist in equal proportions. This would be an explosive combination since, as we have seen, in the presence of iron or copper the two react to produce the hydroxy radical. It is the simultaneous scavenging of hydrogen peroxide by glutathione peroxidase that makes the total process both efficient and safe.

Second, the glutathione system is the only enzyme system to scavenge lipid peroxides.[26] This service is hard to overestimate. Cleaning up lipid peroxide performs three important functions.

1. It prevents the deterioration of lipid peroxide into cross-linking aldehyde.

2. It stops lipid peroxide from interacting with iron or copper in the chain branching reaction that produces two more free radicals—the alkoxy radical and the hydroxy radical.

3. It prevents the chemical reaction which creates chemotactic chemicals to pull in more immune system cells. Reducing this reaction (the *arachidonic acid pathway*) slows the arrival of more free radical-spilling phagocytes, and prevents the creation of free radicals churned out as the chemotactic chemicals are created.

Each time glutathione peroxidase disarms a lipid peroxide molecule, it defuses an explosion of potential damage.

The glutathione system is more complex than SOD and catalase, involving three different enzymes. The glutathione peroxidase enzyme uses a molecule of glutathione as its sword in the anti-free radical fight. It hands an electron from glutathione to hydrogen peroxide or lipid peroxide, thus satisfying their electron hunger and settling them down. The glutathione molecule, then short an electron, must be taken in hand by a second enzyme, glutathione reductase. This enzyme puts an electron back into glutathione, readying it once more for the fight. A third enzyme manufactures the glutathione itself from three amino acid molecules and four selenium atoms. Because all components of this process are at high concentrations in the cell, the process is extremely efficient—as long as there is sufficient selenium to create glutathione (see below).[27]

The glutathione system is a *sine qua non* of human life. In stark contrast to catalase, a hereditary deficiency of glutathione synthetase (the enzyme that creates glutathione) leads to premature death from oxidative damage in the brain.[28] Laboratory work has demonstrated the positive side: administration of glutathione to rats with liver tumors caused regression of tumors in 81% of the experimental group.[29]

Since selenium is an essential component of glutathione, data on selenium intake is another measure of the importance of this anti-oxidant system. The National Research Council has issued an official publication stating that high levels of selenium in the diet or drinking water protect against many types of cancer.[30] Where selenium soil concentrations in America are highest (South Dakota), cancer incidence is lowest. The reverse is true in Ohio, where the lowest levels of selenium correlate with the highest levels of cancer.[31] People with high levels of selenium in the bloodstream also exhibit the fewest cancers.[32] All this evidence indicates that the glutathione system, with four molecules of selenium in each glutathione molecule, strongly inhibits the free radical cascades that attack DNA.

Ingesting selenium also protects the liver against damage from carbon tetrachloride. Since carbon tetrachloride does its damage when broken down into the highly reactive trichloromethyl free radical, this is more evidence that the glutathione system inhibits free radical damage.[33]

As we have seen, lipid peroxide spurs the creation of chemotactic chemicals. One set of these chemicals, the leukotrienes, has been implicated in the stimulation of asthma. Selenium (the glutathione system) may thus be useful in treating asthma.[34] The evidence is persuasive: in great part, human beings owe their lives and health to the constant vigilance of the glutathione anti-oxidant system.

EXTRACELLULAR FREE RADICAL QUENCHERS

In addition to these enzymes which transform free radicals and ROS into less dangerous molecules, the body also has free radical quenchers which offer up electrons to satisfy the free radical thirst. These willing molecules are *endogenous*—created within the body—and they fill a major hole in the body's anti-oxidant defense system. The enzymes we have discussed patrol only within individual cells. This leaves no first-line defense against external attacks on cell membranes. But many of the body's own free radical quenchers are *extracellular*—outside the cells. Most circulate in the bloodstream and diffuse into the spaces between cells, thus providing protection where the enzymes do not.

Uric acid. One of these free radical quenchers is uric acid, or urate. In laboratory tests, uric acid scavenges superoxide as effectively as vitamin C. It also defuses the hydroxy radical, as well as the lipid peroxy radical that first results from free radical attack on the cell membrane. Work by Bruce Ames at the University of California, Berkeley, has shown that uric acid can be present at high levels in the bloodstream, far higher than is common with vitamin C. His work has also shown that red blood cells can take up uric acid from the bloodstream, which helps protect them against lipid peroxidation. Dr. Ames speculates that when human beings lost the ability to synthesize their own vitamin C (see discussion below), uric acid may have stepped in to help fill the gap.[35]

Ceruloplasmin. A second endogenous free radical quencher is known as ceruloplasmin. This protein carries a copper molecule which is willing to give up an electron to quench free radicals. It scavenges superoxide, the hydroxy radical, and singlet oxygen, and it may account for as much as 70% of the anti-oxidant activity in the bloodstream.[36] Levels of ceruloplasmin increase after an injury, indicating it is inducible when needed to fight the excess free radicals produced by inflammation. Ceruloplasmin inhibits cell death during inflammation,[37] and people with rheumatoid arthritis have elevated levels of ceruloplasmin, apparently to fight excess free radical production.[38]

Spare parts. Some free radical researchers consider the cell's spare parts as an aspect of anti-oxidant defense. In this view, if free radicals attack amino acids which have not yet been structured into proteins, or nucleotide bases which have not yet been included in DNA or RNA, this is a net gain for the cell as a whole. Such raw materials are readily available, and the cell has not yet spent the time and energy needed to build them into the critically important macromolecules. If you had to choose between termites in a wood pile and termites in your house, the wood pile would be the logical choice. There is a cost to losing raw materials, but not as great as the cost of losing finished goods.

Iron sequestration. If iron atoms are free and available, they can catalyze the *Fenton reaction*—allowing superoxide and hydrogen peroxide to react, with the hydroxy radical as the lethal result. The body thus attempts to keep a close watch on iron. Once the iron molecule has been encased in an enzyme, most researchers believe it is prevented from doing harm. But iron must be moved in the bloodstream to bring it to the cells for inclusion in enzymes. In a free state it would be dangerous, so it is carried by a protein molecule called transferrin. Like a deputy sheriff transporting a prisoner, transferrin keeps the iron handcuffed and unavailable for reaction. Inside the cell the iron is stored in ferritin molecules, which also keep it out of trouble.[39]

This system is far better than letting iron move freely, but it is not foolproof. The iron must be let loose within the cell eventually so it is available for inclusion in enzymatic molecules. When those enzymes are broken down, as most are within a few days, the iron is set free once again. Free iron floating within the cell, even within the nucleus, is a necessary part of the body's enzyme production—so no system of iron control can ever be 100% effective.

EDIBLE DEFENSE AGAINST FREE RADICALS

The body's endogenous anti-oxidant defenses are varied and impressively effective. It seems clear, however, that they are not sufficient in themselves to maintain a steady state of health—a physical body that does not age or fall ill. The most obvious evidence for this is that people do still age and fall ill.

We have already seen a more statistically rigorous argument: Animals can use their mitochondrial transport chains to burn, on average, only a pre-set number of calories. Human beings have the best anti-oxidant defenses, and can therefore burn four times more calories per pound than, say, a mouse.[40] But limits still exist, meaning that free radical damage still continues. Though the human physiology has made progress toward a balance between anti-oxidants and free radicals, slow motion oxidative stress still seems a reality for even the healthiest people. The free radical clock is still ticking.

These facts have led many in the free radical field to look for ways to supplement human anti-oxidant defenses. The human physiology already stops free radical attacks ten times better than the mouse and the human life span is roughly 30 times longer than the mouse's. What if we could double our anti-oxidant effectiveness? Would life span double as well? Can human beings reach their 150th birthday as routinely as they now reach their 75th?

Many researchers feel such progress is plausible. They base their opinions on an outpouring of research. These studies show that it is definitely possible to augment the body's free radical defense.

One approach is through pharmaceutical agents, known anti-oxidants such as probucol and *N-tert-butyl-alpha-phenylnitrone* (PBN). But as we saw in Part One, all drugs are likely to have side effects, and natural substances are more likely to interact effortlessly with the body's mechanics. Pharmaceutical agents may have their role in a sudden crisis, especially associated with surgery. But as long as plant products are at least as effective as artificial drugs, it seems logical to stay with the natural approach. And as we will see in the next chapter, natural herbal formulas can actually scavenge free radicals much more effectively than pharmaceuticals.

In the realm of natural substances, many edible nutrients have been shown to quench free radicals, slow the aging process, and prevent the most serious degenerative diseases. These substances are effective and side effects are minimal.

Vitamin C. The most famous of the nutrient anti-oxidants is doubtless vitamin C. Nobel laureate Linus Pauling spent long years trying to convince the medical establishment that vitamin C had therapeutic effects. Now the free radical research has belatedly shown him right.

Vitamin C is water soluble. It is found inside the cell in the aqueous cytosol, and also in the bloodstream and intercellular spaces. It is found in high concentrations in the lung (where there are high levels of oxygen) and especially in the brain (where, researchers speculate, it may protect neurotransmitter chemicals from free radical damage as they are being sent from one nerve to the next).[41]

Vitamin C scavenges superoxide, though not as well as the enzyme SOD. Unlike any enzyme, however, vitamin C can quench the hydroxy radical directly.[42] It also scavenges singlet oxygen.[43] Low levels of vitamin C in the blood correlate with bladder cancer.[44] When laboratory animals are given a dose of vitamin C corresponding to a human dose of 1.5 grams per day, it helps prevent these bladder tumors.[45] Many other studies have also shown that vitamin C helps inhibit cancer,[46] including a famous study by Dr. Pauling showing that severe cancer patients treated with vitamin C lived an average of 300 days longer than patients who did not receive vitamin C.[47] The Mayo Clinic subsequently tried vitamin C with cancer patients, and failed to replicate these results—a result the media widely publicized. Dr. Pauling pointed out a simple reason for this failure to replicate. Vitamin C lasts only four to six hours in the bloodstream before it is cleared. He therefore gave his patients vitamin C in divided doses several times a day. The Mayo Clinic gave only one large daily dose, meaning the patients were unprotected for at least 18 hours out of 24.[48]

The many studies indicating vitamin C inhibits cancer are consistent with its known ability to scavenge free radicals—especially the hydroxy radical. Researchers have also found that use of vitamin C as an adjunct to radiation therapy appears to reduce collateral damage to healthy tissue—a result consistent with its ability to scavenge free radicals.[49] There is also evidence that vitamin C reduces free radical damage during inflammation, thereby reducing the inflammation itself.[50] Studies have also shown that vitamin C speeds recovery from heart attacks.[51] White blood cells rush vitamin C to the heart after a heart attack, even if they have to seriously deplete vitamin C levels in other organs.[52] Since injured areas attract neutrophils and macrophages, with their profligate free radical ways, it is likely the increased vitamin C helps keep the inevitable damage under control. Vitamin C also reduces platelet aggregation and blood clotting.[53]

Given these wide-ranging anti-oxidant benefits, it is interesting that about 250,000 years ago the human body lost its ability to produce vitamin C. Most animals create their own, and a 150-pound animal typically makes about ten grams of vitamin C per day (the equivalent of about 100 large glasses of orange juice). When under stress, moreover, animals greatly increase their production of vitamin C—to fight the free radicals that stress creates.[54] There is a cost to this vitamin C production, however. Animals make vitamin C in the liver by converting glucose. Some researchers feel that, by giving up this internal production of vitamin C, the human being had more glucose to deal with sudden emergency requirements for energy.

We have seen that the body produces uric acid, ceruloplasmin, and other endogenous free radical quenchers, perhaps to fill the void created by the lost ability to make vitamin C. But some clinicians, led by Dr. Robert V. Cathcart, believe that vitamin C should still be taken in what other medical experts consider very high doses. Dr. Cathcart recommends 10 to 15 grams a day when healthy, and 50 grams or more per day when sick. Since excess vitamin C produces diarrhea, Dr. Cathcart recommends taking a dosage just below this limit. His most convincing point is that during illness, when free radical damage caused by the immune system is high, people can absorb much higher levels of vitamin C without suffering diarrhea. Vitamin C is apparently used up in the free radical battle.[55]

Taking high levels of vitamin C by itself, however, bears some resemblance to taking prescription drugs. In both cases, a single type of molecule is being ingested in large quantities. The chance for side effects is high. For example, people who have a propensity for the creation of oxalic acid (oxalate) kidney stones are at risk when taking vitamin C.[56] Under stress, large amounts of vitamin C can actually help *create* free radicals.[57] Administering vitamin C with a magic bullet mentality may not be its best use.

Vitamin E. While vitamin C goes on patrol in aqueous regions, the fat-soluble anti-oxidant vitamin E takes up its station in lipid membranes of the cell. It is found in all cell membranes, including the outer cell membrane, the endoplasmic reticulum, and the inner and outer membranes of the mitochondria.[58]

Vitamin E acts as a first, fast-reacting defense against free radical damage to the membrane lipids. As soon as a lipid has been attacked and radicalized (turned into a lipid peroxy radical), vitamin E intervenes by sacrificing an electron. This satisfies the peroxy radical and prevents it from stealing an electron from a neighboring molecule in the lipid bilayer— thus blocking the free radical chain reaction from rolling destructively down the membrane.[59] But this gallant act by vitamin E still turns the peroxy radical into lipid peroxide— which, though relatively stable, has the destructive future we described previously. Thus, vitamin E works in conjunction with glutathione peroxidase. Vitamin E stops the peroxy radical chain reaction. The lipid peroxide left behind is scavenged by the glutathione system.

Researchers estimate that a single molecule of vitamin E within a membrane is sufficient to protect 1000 lipid molecules from the free radical chain reaction. If vitamin E is low, lipid peroxidation increases. If vitamin E does not stop the chain reaction from rolling down the cell membrane, one lipid peroxide is left behind for every former membrane lipid—and the challenge to glutathione peroxidase is much greater.[60]

Vitamin E also stops lung damage caused by air pollution. Though nitrogen dioxide and ozone are free radicals and set off free radical chain reactions, vitamin E can stop the reactions. This prevents lipid peroxide molecules from being created in large numbers—reducing the number that can degenerate into aldehyde. The lungs are thereby protected from cross-linking damage.[61] Like the glutathione enzyme system, vitamin E also prevents damage to the liver when carbon tetrachloride is transformed into the trichloromethyl free radical.[62]

Vitamin E has long been known for its ability to increase strength and endurance, and this now seems to be explained by its anti-oxidant capabilities. When the body exercises, it burns more fuel, racing the mitochondrial electron transport chain and creating more free radicals. These free radicals can create more membrane damage, especially in the mitochondria itself—restricting energy production. Not only could the membrane work surface be degraded, but the electron transport enzymes themselves could be damaged when the chain of free radical damage reaches them. A number of studies have shown that vitamin E protects against the creation of excess lipid peroxide during physical exercise.[63] Endurance markedly improves.[64] No studies more clearly show the ongoing destruction caused by the free radical toxic waste in the cell's energy plants—and the possibility for bringing such damage under control.

Vitamin E also reduces atherosclerosis and formation of blood clots in blood vessels by cutting off free radical chain reactions in cell membranes and thus preventing damage to artery linings and excess lipid peroxidation. It helps prevent deep vein clots, even in postoperative patients who must remain immobile for long periods of time.[65] Vitamin E also ameliorates several circulatory conditions, including heart disease.[66] In addition, vitamin E can powerfully protect against the free radical damage caused during heart bypass surgery. Fourteen patients who took 300 milligrams of vitamin E every day for two weeks prior to their surgery showed a marked improvement in the heart's ability to pump normally during the crucial first five hours after surgery.[67]

Vitamin E is not known for negative side effects, though it may cause a slight rise in blood pressure when first taken.[68] The only limitation of vitamin E is one that is typical of all nutrient anti-oxidants: Once it has made its sacrificial electron donation to a free radical, it becomes stale. It can't work usefully again without picking up a replacement electron.

Beta-carotene. In addition to vitamins C and E, a third micronutrient has been thoroughly researched. This is beta-carotene, the substance that gives carrots their color. Beta-carotene is a precursor of vitamin A; the body converts it to vitamin A in the small intestine. Vitamin A has some toxic effects in large doses, but regardless of how much beta-carotene is taken in, the body will never itself create excess vitamin A. Thus, beta-carotene appears to be the safest way to take vitamin A.[69] Moreover, excess beta-carotene, over and above the amount needed to create vitamin A, has a well-documented ability to fight cancer—with no toxic side effects at any dosage.[70]

Beta-carotene is the most efficient quencher of singlet oxygen known, thus filling a hole in the enzyme defenses.[71] It also works effectively against many other free radicals and ROS,[72] and is fat-soluble, allowing it to work in tandem with vitamin E in lipid membranes of the cell.[73]

Beta-carotene is especially effective against cancer.[74] Dr. Eli Seifter of the Albert Einstein College of Medicine in New York has demonstrated that when laboratory animals with cancer were given beta-carotene along with radiation therapy, the therapy was much more effective.[75] Researchers at Johns Hopkins School of Hygiene and Public Health have discovered that people with low levels of beta-carotene in the bloodstream are roughly four times more likely to develop a common form of lung cancer.[76]

As with all anti-oxidants that protect against cancer, these findings also indicate that beta-carotene may retard the aging process. Cancer can result when free radicals attack the DNA. But attacks on DNA can also hit genes in the *major histocompatibility complex* (MHC) that regulate SOD and the glutathione system, thus weakening the body's response to free radicals. Attacks at many places on the DNA can result in less effective functioning and dysdifferentiation. As Richard Cutler of the National Institute of Aging says, the longevity of an animal "may be governed in part by the same mechanisms as those processes governing species' differences in their age-dependent probability of developing cancer."[77] Any anti-oxidant that protects DNA from cancer-causing damage most likely protects it against the aging process as well.

Bioflavonoids. Many other natural substances have anti-oxidant effects. As a general statement, most plants are richly endowed with anti-oxidants. Plants are bathed in the sun's radiation and generate high levels of oxygen as a by-product of photosynthesis. Anywhere there is radiation plus oxygen, free radicals and ROS are bound to be created in profusion. Plants must load up with anti-oxidants to deal with the fall-out.

Hundreds of these plant compounds are known by the general label *polyphenols*. The largest and most thoroughly researched subgroup of polyphenols is known as the *bioflavonoids*. These natural substances create the beautiful deep blues and reds in fruits, berries, and wine. They are often tart and bitter to the taste, but can also be sweet. When you smell the rich aroma of coffee, or enjoy the smooth taste of vanilla ice cream, you are encountering polyphenol molecules. They put the kick in red peppers and protect our foods from going stale from oxygen damage.

All these substances have basic molecular similarities, but the hundreds of variations produce a rich variety of effects. It is only in recent years that the complexities of their benefits have begun to be defined through systematic research. In fact, some early researchers in the free radical field dismissed bioflavonoids as insignificant. This was especially true of scientists who favored artificial vitamins. To them, a vitamin is a single, isolated molecule which can (frequently) be duplicated in the laboratory. In this vitamin version of the magic bullet approach, vitamin C is an "active ingredient." All the hundreds of extra molecular types that come trailing along with the natural vitamin C from an orange are considered extraneous.[78] However, laboratory investigation has made this view obsolete. Polyphenols in general, and bioflavonoids in particular, have now become leading subjects in free radical research. Plants are very good at creating anti-oxidants. It is simply taking researchers a long time to identify the wide variety.

Bioflavonoid research was begun in 1928, quite by accident, by the European scientist Dr. Szent-Gyorgi—who had already secured his place in nutritional history with the discovery of ascorbic acid (vitamin C). A friend of Dr. Szent-Gyorgi's was suffering from bleeding gums. Since bleeding gums are one symptom of scurvy (a vitamin C deficiency disease), Dr. Szent-Gyorgi decided to give his friend some ascorbic acid. The only supply he had was not yet purified; it was still "tainted" with many natural compounds. Dr. Szent-Gyorgi decided impure vitamin C was better than none at all, and sure enough, his friend got well. Surprisingly, subsequent tests with pure vitamin C failed to produce any benefit. Dr. Szent-Gyorgi then withheld the vitamin C and instead gave the "contaminants." The gums healed perfectly. A new class of bioactive molecules had been discovered.

As with much else in natural medicine, however, mainstream medical investigators paid scant attention. Half a century passed before the undertaking of a serious research effort on polyphenols and bioflavonoids—but now the data are copious and impressive. Many bioflavonoids scavenge free radicals, and some chelate metals (tying them up so they can't react with oxygen). As a result, they produce positive effects on many disease conditions.

Many bioflavonoids have been tested for their ability to stop membrane-destroying lipid peroxidation. A number of studies have demonstrated that two bioflavonoids in particular—quercetin and catechin—produce a potent protective effect. Others, such as morin, rutin, and naringin are also protective, but less so.[79]

Other studies show that quercetin, rutin, morin, and other bioflavonoids inhibit free radical creation during the inflammatory reaction by inhibiting the production of leukotrienes—the chemotactic messengers that summon white blood cells.[80] The first study showing that bioflavonoids can actually reduce inflammation appeared in 1971. Since then, research has shown that procyanidin (from grapes),[81] anthocyanins (from the bilberry),[82] and other bioflavonoids inhibit excessive inflammation in animals. The results are sometimes striking; hyoplaetin reduces inflammatory swelling in mice by as much as 75%.[83]

Bioflavonoids also fight cancer—in both the initiation and promotion phases. Many cancer studies have shown that bioflavonoids can reduce the incidence of cancer in animals.[84] Also, researchers often assess the effectiveness of a given substance by checking for *dose dependence*—increasing benefit from increasing doses; one study showed that quercetin's anticancer effects were dose dependent all the way up to 5% of the diet, a figure unusually high.[85]

Researchers attribute most of this anti-cancer effect to bioflavonoids' anti-oxidant qualities. But two studies have demonstrated an additional effect of great significance. Some bioflavonoids potentiate the activity of enzymes which destroy or neutralize carcinogenic substances.[86] Research on such enzyme effects are just beginning, but it is an area of great promise.

Not surprisingly, bioflavonoids also slow the development of cardiovascular disease. To begin with, several bioflavonoids reduce overall levels of circulating lipids in the bloodstream.[87]

Of those tested, the most effective was tannic acid, a component of many popular beverages. Quercetin, morin, and fisetin also inhibit the formation of the dangerous LDL-ox.[88] Bioflavonoids seem well-suited to prevention of the membrane damage typical of atherosclerosis because they can situate themselves comfortably within the lipid bilayer and offer immediate protection. In such a strategic position, they can not only stop free radical attack themselves, but also pass an electron to stale vitamin E, putting that membrane protector back in the fight.[89]

In addition to the health-promoting effects typical of antioxidants, bioflavonoids also exhibit wide-ranging serendipity that can be so useful in naturally occurring nutrients. We have already seen that they can enliven certain enzyme systems in the body. Some bioflavonoids can also fight bacteria and viruses directly. It has long been known that some food plants have antibacterial properties. Cranberries, for example, have frequently been recommended by nurses to counteract urinary infection—though the mechanisms weren't understood.

Now research indicates that most of the natural antimicrobial activity in the plant kingdom is due to bioflavonoids. The antibacterial qualities in cranberries, for example, have been attributed to the action of proanthocyanidins and flavonols.[90] Another study showed that biflavanones from a traditional African medicinal herb inhibited bacterial growth in both tissue cultures and animals.[91] Quercetin, luteolin, morin, fisetin, procyanidin, and other bioflavonoids also inhibit the activity of a variety of viruses.[92]

Finally, the most thoroughly researched health benefit of bioflavonoids is their ability to reduce allergies and asthma. This is partly because they block the release of histamines, which stimulate the allergic reaction, and partly because they block leukotriene synthesis, slowing the inflammatory reaction.[93] There is no longer any doubt that bioflavonoids help control free radicals and promote health in many ways.

CAN WE MAXIMIZE FREE RADICAL DEFENSE?

A short summary of this chapter: The body has its own free radical-fighting systems—and we can effectively supplement these systems with edible nutrients. The body's anti-oxidant enzymes, especially SOD and the glutathione system, are alert and effective within the cell. Circulating biochemicals such as uric acid and ceruloplasmin take the battle out into the inter-cellular spaces and bloodstream. Vitamins C and E, beta-carotene, and bioflavonoids all add significantly to the anti-free radical forces—both inside and outside the cells.

It obviously makes sense to bolster our free radical defenses. But finding the most effective system for ingesting these molecular reinforcements is a challenge. It's true that eating a healthy diet that includes fruits and vegetables can provide vitamins and other anti-oxidants. However, most people don't eat a healthy diet. Moreover, many free radical researchers believe that anti-oxidants must be taken in doses far more concentrated than those found in even a normal healthy diet.

In fact, the free radical research has added a new approach to good nutrition. It is one thing to take in enough vitamins and minerals to make the major systems of the body function correctly. This type of nutritional need is theoretically identified in the Recommended Daily Allowances published by the federal government. But anti-oxidants cannot be confused with these basic nutritional needs. Anti-oxidants are not taken for their use in the cell's ordinary housekeeping. Anti-oxidants are taken to fight off the constant waves of free radicals. For this purpose, research makes it seem likely that we must either take far larger doses of some vitamins than we have previously thought necessary, or else find a new and more effective source of anti-oxidant defense.

Direct consumption of enzymes is not the answer. They are far more powerful than vitamins and other nutrients, but as we saw in Part One, enzymes cannot be taken by mouth. They are gigantic protein molecules that cannot pass through the walls of the digestive system and into the bloodstream. Digestive juices break them down into their component amino acids, a pile of generic building blocks. It's true that SOD has been given by injection directly into inflamed joints, but this is not a practical program for home use.

What is the optimal anti-oxidant approach? A hint is provided by much of the research on vitamins and other such nutrients: Anti-oxidants tend to work synergistically. Just as glutathione reductase puts an electron back into stale glutathione, allowing it to be used again to donate that electron to a free radical, so ingested anti-oxidants also tend to recycle each other. If a vitamin E molecule has spent its available electron to stop a free radical chain reaction, vitamin C can replace that electron. When vitamin C gets short, bioflavonoids and various components of vitamin B can be of help. Glutathione can also recharge both vitamins C and E—as long as there is sufficient selenium.[94] And many of these anti-oxidants, such as vitamin C and bioflavonoids, not only fight free radicals but also contribute to good health in other ways.

The body faces a mortal challenge in oxidative stress. Anti-oxidant forces tend to work together to meet that challenge. The question is how this natural teamwork can be maximized. It is time to investigate ancient anti-oxidant formulations intended to make optimal use of nature's synergism.

Notes

1. Ames BN, Shigenaga MK, "DNA Damage by Endogenous Oxidants and Mitogenesis As Causes of Aging and Cancer" in *Molecular Biology of Free Radical Scavenging Systems*, Scandalios JG, ed. (Cold Spring Harbor Laboratory Press, Plainview, 1992), pp. 1-21

2. Kronhausen E, et al, *Formula for Life* (William Morrow and Company, New York, 1989), p. 77

3. Richards RT, Sharma HM, *Indian J Clin Prac* 2(1991): 15-26

4. Gregory EM, Fridovich I, *J Bacteriol* 114(1973): 543-8

5. Krinsky NI, "Biological Roles of Singlet Oxygen" in *Singlet Oxygen*, Wasserman HH, Murray RW, eds. (Academic Press, New York, 1979), pp. 597-641; Singh A, et al, *Bull Europ Physiopath Resp* 17(1981)(Supplement): 31-41; Singh A, *Can J Physiol Pharmacol* 60(1982): 1330-45

6. Levine SA, Kidd PM, *Antioxidant Adaptation: Its Role in Free Radical Pathology* (Biocurrents Division, Allergy Research Group, San Leandro, 1986), p. 49

7. Richards, *Indian* (see note 3)

8. Niwa Y, Tsutsui D, *Saishinigaku (Japan)* 38(1983): 1450-8

9. Fridovich I, "Superoxide Dismutase in Biology and Medicine" in *Pathology of Oxygen*, Autor AP, ed. (Academic Press, New York, 1982), pp. 1-19

10. Tanaka K, Sugahara K, *Plant Cell Physiol* 21(1980): 601-11; Rabinowitch HD, et al, *Arch Biochem Biophys* 225(1983): 640-8

11. Niwa, *Saishinigaku* (see note 8)

12. Forman HJ, Fisher AB, *Lab Invest* 45(1981): 1-6; Steinberg H, et al, *Am Rev Respir Dis* 128(1983): 94-7; Fantone JC, Ward PA, *Current Concepts: Oxygen-Derived Radicals and Their Metabolites: Relationship to Tissue Injury* (The Upjohn Company, Kalamazoo, 1985), p. 43

13. Freeman BA, et al, *J Biol Chem* 258(1983): 12534-42

14. Crapo JD, McCord JM, *Am J Physiol* 231(1976): 1196-1203

15. Petrone WF, et al, *Proc Natl Acad Sci USA* 77(1980): 1159-63; Perez HD, et al, *Inflammation* 4(1980): 313-28

16. Niwa Y, et al, *Life Sci* 40(1987): 921-7; Niwa Y, et al, *Life Sci* 42(1988): 351-6

17. Sugiura K, et al, *Jap J Dermatol (Japan)* 96(1986): 171-4

18. Niwa, *Life* (see note 16)

19. Fridovich I, "Oxygen Radicals, Hydrogen Peroxide, and Oxygen Toxicity" in *Free Radicals in Biology, Vol. 1*, Pryor WA, ed. (Academic Press, New York, 1976), pp. 239-77

20. de Duve C, *A Guided Tour of the Living Cell, Vol. 1*, (Scientific American Library, New York, 1984), pp. 180-7

21. Cutler RG, *Am J Clin Nutr* 53(1991): 373S-9S

22. Aebi E, Wyss SR, "Acatalasemia" in *The Metabolic Basis of Inherited Disease (5th Edition)* Stanbury JB, et al, eds. (McGraw-Hill, New York, 1983), pp. 1421-2

23. Larsson A, et al, eds., *Functions of Glutathione: Biochemical, Physiological, Toxicological, and Clinical Aspects* (Raven Press, New York, 1983)

24. Levine, *Antioxidant* (see note 6), pp. 50-1

25. Fridovich, "Oxygen" (see note 19)

26. Farber J, et al, *Lab Invest* 62(1990): 670-9

27. Larsson, *Functions* (see note 23)

28. Ibid

29. Novi AM, *Science* 212(1981): 541-2

30. *Diet, Nutrition, and Cancer* (National Academy Press, Washington, D.C., 1982)

31. Shamberger RJ, et al, *Arch Environ Health* 31(1976): 231-5; Schrauzer GN, et al, *Bioinorg Chem* 7(1977): 23-31; Schrauzer GN, et al, *Bioinorg Chem* 8(1978): 303-18; Mondragon MC, Jaffe WG, *Arch Latinoamer Nutr* 26(1976): 341-52

32. Salonen JT, et al, *Brit Med J* 290(1985): 417-20

33. Hafeman DG, Hoekstra WG, *J Nutr* 107(1977): 656-65; Ibid, pp. 666-72

34. McCarty M, *Med Hypoth* 13(1984): 45-50

35. Ames BN, et al, *Proc Natl Acad Sci USA* 78(1981): 6858-62

36. Levine, *Antioxidant* (see note 6), p. 60

37. Lvstad RA, *Int J Biochem* 13(1981): 221-4; Denko CW, *Agents Actions* 9(1979): 333-6

38. Halliwell B, *Bull Europ Physiopath Resp* 17(1981)(Supplement): 21-9; Dormandy TL, "Ceruloplasmin and Serum Antioxidant Activity" in *Oxygen Free Radicals and Tissue Damage*, Gilbert DL, ed. (Excerpta Medica, New York, 1979), pp. 166-8

39. Cotran RS, et al, eds., *Robbins Pathologic Basis of Disease* (W.B. Saunders Co., Philadelphia, 1989), pp. 25-6, 686-8

40. Cutler, *Am J* (see note 21)

41. Ibid; Willis RJ, Kratzing CC, *Biochem Biophys Res Comm* 59(1974): 1250-2

42. Florence TM, *Int Clin Nutr Rev* 4(1984): 6-19

43. Bendich A, et al, *Adv Free Radic Biol Med* 2(1986): 419-44

44. Schlegel JU, et al, *J Urol* 97(1967): 479-81

45. Schlegel JU, et al, *J Urol* 103(1970): 155-9

46. Graham S, et al, *Am J Epidem* 113(1981): 675-7

47. Pauling L, *How to Live Longer and Feel Better* (W.H. Freeman & Company, New York, 1986), pp. 173-9

48. Ibid

49. Cheraskin E, et al, *Acta Cytologica* 12(1968): 433-8

50. Beisel WR, *Am J Clin Nutr* 35(Supplement)(1982): 417-68

51. Kronhausen, *Formula* (see note 2), p. 103

52. Hume R, et al, *Brit Heart J* 34(1972): 238-43

53. Spittle CR, *Lancet* 2(1973): 199-201 (letter); Sarji KE, et al, *Thrombosis Research* 15(1979): 639-50; Bordia AK, *Atherosclerosis* 35(1980): 181-7; Cardova C, et al, *Atherosclerosis* 41(1982):15-9

54. Kronhausen, *Formula* (see note 2), p. 96

55. Levine, *Antioxidant* (see note 6), pp. 308-11

56. Kronhausen, *Formula* (see note 2), p. 105

57. Niwa Y, et al, *Drugs Exp Clin Res* XIV(1988): 361-72; Dormandy T, *Lancet* 1(1978): 647-50

58. Machin J, Bendich A, *FASEB J* 1(1987): 441

59. Diplock AT, *Am J Clin Nutr* 53(1991): 189S-93S; Niki E, et al, *Am J Clin Nutr* 53(1991): 201S-5S; Di Mascio P, et al, *Am J Clin Nutr* 53(1991): 194S-200S

60. Forman HJ, Fisher AB, "Antioxidant Defenses" in *Oxygen and Living Processes*, Gilbert DL, ed. (Springer-Verlag, New York, 1981), pp. 235-72; Lubin B, Machlin LJ, eds. "Vitamin E: Biochemical, Hematological, and Clinical Aspects" *New York Academy of Sciences, Annals, Vol. 393* (1982)

61. Roehm JN, et al, *Arch Environ Health* 24(1972): 237-42; Mustafa MG, *Nutr Rep Int* 11(1975): 475-81; Fletcher BL, Tappel AL, *Environ Res* 6(1973): 165-75

62. Butler TC, *J Pharmacol Exp Ther* 134(1961): 311-9

63. Tappel AL, "Measurement of and Protection From in Vivo Lipid Peroxidation" in *Free Radicals in Biology, Vol. IV*, Pryor WA, ed.

(Academic Press, New York, 1980), pp. 1-47; Dillard CJ, et al, *J Appl Physiol* 45(1978): 927-32

64. Davies KJ, et al, *Biochem Biophys Res Comm* 107(1982): 1198-205

65. Ochsner A, et al, *JAMA* 144(1950): 831-4; Ochsner A, *N Eng J Med* 271(1964): 211 (letter)

66. Shute WE, Taub HJ, *Vitamin E for Ailing and Healthy Hearts* (Pyramid House, New York, 1969)

67. Fackelmann KA, *Sci News* 138(1990): 333

68. Kronhausen, *Formula* (see note 2), p. 112

69. Ibid, pp. 115-16

70. Ibid, p. 114

71. Diplock, *Am J* (see note 59)

72. Di Mascio, *Am J* (see note 59)

73. Burton GW, Ingold KU, *Science* 224(1984): 569-73

74. Peto R, et al, *Nature* 290(1981): 201-8

75. Hendler SS, *The Complete Guide to Anti-Aging Nutrients* (Simon and Schuster, New York, 1984), p. 88; Harris RWC, *Brit J Cancer* 53(1986): 653-9; Shekelle RB, et al, *Lancet* 2(1981): 1185-90

76. Menkes MS, et al, *N Eng J Med* 315(1986): 1250-89

77. Cutler RG, *Proc Natl Acad Sci USA* 81(1984): 7629-31

78. Kronhausen, *Formula* (see note 2), p. 106

79 Affany A, et al, *Fund Clin Pharmacol* 1(1987): 451-7; Das N, Ratty A, "Effects of Flavonoids on Induced Non-Enzymatic Lipid Peroxidation" in *Plant Flavonoids In Biology and Medicine, Vol. 1* (Alan R. Liss, Inc., New York, 1986), pp. 243-7

80. Baumann J, et al, *Prostaglandins* 20(1980): 627-39; Hsieh R, et al, *Lipids* 23(1988): 322-6

81. Blazso G, Gabor M, *Acta Physiol Acad Sci (Hungary)* 56(1980): 235-40

82. Lietti A, et al, *Arzneimittel-Forschung (Drug Research)* 26(1976): 829-33

83. Villar A, et al, *J Pharmacy Pharmacol* 36(1984): 820-3

84. Wattenberg L, Leong J, *Can Res* 30(1970): 1922-5; Marwan A, Nagel C, *J Food Sci* 51(1986): 1009-13; Shamberger R, *Nutrition and Cancer* (Plenum Press, New York, 1984); Bracke M, et al, "Flavonoids Inhibit Malignant Tumor Invasion In Vitro" in *Plant Flavonoids In Biology and Medicine, Vol. 2*(Alan R. Liss, Inc., New York, 1988), pp. 219-33

85. Yasukawa K, et al, "Effect of Flavonoids On Tumor Promoter's Activity" in *Plant Flavonoids In Biology and Medicine, Vol. 2* (Alan R. Liss, Inc., New York, 1988), pp. 247-50

86. Wattenberg, *Can* (see note 84); Kuttan R, et al, *Experientia* 37(1981): 221-3

87. Yugarani T, et al, *Lipids* 27(1992): 181-6

88. Whalley CV, et al, *Biochem Pharmacol* 39(1990): 1743-50

89. Leibovitz BE, *Nutrition Update* 6(1992): 1-15

90. Marwan, *J Food* (see note 84)

91. Iwu M, "Biflavanones of Garcinia: Pharmacological and Biological Activities" in *Plant Flavonoids In Biology and Medicine, Vol. 1* (Alan R. Liss, Inc., New York, 1986), pp. 485-8

92. Beladi I, et al, *Ann NY Acad Sci* 284(1977): 358-64

93. Saylor B, *Arch Otolaryngol* 50(1949): 813-20; Schoenkerman B, Justice R, *Ann Allergy* 10(1952): 138-41

94. Kronhausen, *Formula* (see note 2), pp. 91-118

CHAPTER FIVE

The Natural Solution to Free Radicals

What we have seen so far is hopeful. It is true that free radicals are wildly destructive. But their damage can be controlled. In the earliest atomic reactors, scientists inserted rods into the radioactive pile (by hand!) to absorb careening neutrons and damp the nuclear reaction. Similarly, we have seen that vitamins, bioflavonoids, and other nutrients can be inserted into the physiology to scavenge free radicals and damp their cell-damaging reactions.

Though the effect of these natural nutrients is encouraging, we have also seen that—molecule for molecule—some of the body's natural enzymes are much more effective. When a molecule of vitamin C or E sacrifices an electron to appease a free radical, the vitamin molecule becomes damaged and useless. Only if it is regenerated by a helpful companion can it reenter the fray. Enzymes, however, can run through thousands of destructive free radicals and ROS without help and without pause.

In an ideal world, therefore, we would find anti-oxidant substances with (1) a low molecular weight, so they can slip from the digestive tract to the bloodstream undamaged, and

(2) the anti-free radical ability, weight for weight, of an enzyme like SOD. It may sound too much to hope for. But if found, such powerful anti-oxidants might tip the scales against free radical damage decisively.

Fortunately, research has identified just such powerful free radical scavengers. This is the research that has changed my career and my life. The studies have shown that certain natural anti-oxidants scavenge superoxide as effectively as SOD. Weight for weight, they stop lipid peroxide chain reactions hundreds and even thousands of times better than anti-oxidant vitamins and a much-researched anti-oxidant drug. They are food supplements. They can be eaten and digested easily. They are the products that interested me in free radical research to begin with—herbal food supplements which are part of Maharishi Ayur-Ved. Modern medical research has discovered the challenge of free radicals. According to many studies, the most effective response comes from the world's oldest system of natural health care.

AN ANCIENT DISCOVERY

As we shall see, these herbal supplements have great promise. Much about them, however, makes experts in Western medical science uneasy. They are not artificial drugs isolated in a test tube. They are natural herbal mixtures from India's Vedic tradition that contain a rich variety of plant substances.

The recipes for these herbal formulations were first discovered thousands of years ago. As with much else in the ancient Vedic tradition, over the course of time knowledge of these herbal supplements was lost to the general public. The herbal formulas were carefully maintained, however, guarded and handed down through generations by a small number of ayurvedic vaidyas.

In 1985, Maharishi Mahesh Yogi met with a number of the leading ayurvedic vaidyas of our time. Maharishi had spent nearly thirty years teaching Transcendental Meditation around the world. Scientific research had validated the effectiveness of this ancient Vedic technique, and the personal experience of millions had indicated that Vedic knowledge could be useful to people in every culture, religion, and walk of life. Now Maharishi was looking for additional knowledge from the Vedic tradition to make available to the modern world. He asked the vaidyas: What more can be done to eliminate disease and suffering?

Among the vaidyas present as Maharishi asked this question, three were most distinguished. The first was Dr. B.D. Triguna, then President of the All-India Ayurveda Congress and Director of the National Academy for Ayurveda, Government of India. The second was the late Dr. V.M. Dwivedi, Professor Emeritus, Gujarat Ayurvedic University and former Vice-Chairman of the Indian government's Ayurveda Pharmacopoeia Committee. Dr. Dwivedi was one of the few remaining vaidyas in India who was a master of the procedures for creating *rasayanas*—herbal formulations that stimulate overall health. The third vaidya was Dr. Balraj Maharshi, an advisor on ayurveda to the government of Andhra Pradesh, India, and perhaps the world's leading expert in Dravyaguna, the identification and utilization of medicinal plants.

It was Dr. Balraj Maharshi who first stepped forward with a specific suggestion. Many years earlier he had studied with a venerable vaidya who had passed on to him the ancient formula for Amrit Kalash—with the admonition that it should only be brought out when the time had come that it could be widely used. After saving the formula for many years, this great expert in plants and herbal formulations decided that Maharishi's worldwide efforts gave Amrit Kalash the opportunity for acceptance around the world. He shared the formula and Maharishi asked him to work with Dr. Triguna, Dr. Dwivedi, and other vaidyas to restore the mixture and its preparation to the high standards of ancient times recorded in the classical ayurvedic texts.

THE TRADITIONAL APPROACH

The results of this cooperative effort have been available in the West for more than five years. Maharishi Amrit Kalash (MAK) is actually composed of two separate formulations. One of these, MAK-4, is an herbal fruit concentrate; the other, MAK-5, is an herbal tablet. Between the two of them, they comprise 24 different herbs and fruits. Each herb and fruit by itself is composed of hundreds, even thousands, of chemical substances—separate types of molecules. Taken together, the mixtures are richly varied.

Traditionally, ayurvedic herbs were prepared through a long and careful process of delicate grinding. The goal was to reduce each component of a formula to the finest possible powder, and no effort was spared to reach this highly refined stage. Modern research has given the explanation for this method of preparation. In a complex natural product, many of the important components are tangled together and unassimilable. The refined grinding process of ayurveda apparently works to enhance digestibility of the various components.

This whole process of formulation and preparation is another aspect of Maharishi Amrit Kalash that is disconcerting to many Western scientists. Those of us who do medical research aren't used to taking whole flowers, plants, and roots and grinding them down into an unanalyzed *potpourri* of various substances. Rather, we are used to seeking for a single active ingredient, a magic bullet to fire at each disease. We are also accustomed to the protocols of objective investigation—taking isolated substances made of identical molecules, testing them in the laboratory, putting them through human clinical trials, and finally prescribing them as cures for specific diseases.

The ancient herbal food supplements from Maharishi Ayur-Ved are completely different. They are compilations of intact plants or parts of plants. They comprise a profusion of components, a rich stew of molecules intended to enrich the human physiology in its entirety. There is no attempt to isolate individual molecules—and these supplements are in no sense drugs. Rather, they are rich herbal foods used as supplements to the everyday diet and said to produce overall health and well-being. Although there have been thousands of years of what we would now call "clinical trials"—systematic use by doctors in their practice—there has not been (until recent years) the type of lab work and systematic experimentation typical of modern medicine. Despite this background, recent scientific experiments have shown these formulas to be dramatically effective—with virtually no side effects.

Why should such an ancient, pre-scientific process yield such impressive scientific effects? Ayurvedic vaidyas assert that the effectiveness of these herbal formulations comes precisely from the richness of their mixtures. They are a deliberate attempt to maximize synergism, the vaidyas maintain; the components help each other move through the digestive system, arrive at the correct cells, penetrate the cell membrane, and achieve intracellular effects.

SCIENCE AND SYNERGISM

Recent research on vitamins and bioflavonoids has identified simple synergistic effects. But assertions about complex synergisms are essentially impossible to check through objective science. In fact, the concept of the isolated active ingredient sprang up largely because modern scientific investigation works best in the simplest situations. It must use a fragmentary, reductionist approach. One aim of scientific investigation is to work on the simplest possible isolated systems.

This approach has a logical basis. With only one type of molecule to work with, a scientist can clearly show cause-and-effect relationships. If you put one type of molecule into your beaker filled with fluid and the fluid turns from colorless to green, you know what caused the change. If you put in two types of molecules and the fluid turns green, you can't be sure if it was one molecule or the other, or a combination of both. The uncertainty increases exponentially as you add more ingredients. Thus, the objective, scientific approach to knowledge biases investigators toward uncomplicated, isolated, reductionist solutions. Science tends to yield simple answers. Scientists look for active ingredients because they can.

Researchers long schooled in this reductionist approach feel uncomfortable when a complex formula such as Maharishi Amrit Kalash is shown to produce positive results. They can hardly resist asking, "Fine, but what ingredient causes the effect?" Their objective training makes it difficult to think holistically, to even consider that it might be all the ingredients at once, working together. They know they will never be able to unravel such complications in the lab. And the tendency is to think, if you can't examine it through reductionist experiment, then it's not significant.

Yet there is no logical reason why substances composed of a single molecular type should be more effective than a carefully chosen combination of ingredients. There is nothing absurd about the idea that a combination of ingredients may produce synergistic effects that enhance effectiveness and reduce side effects. In fact, this view seems to fit naturally with the inconceivably complex operation of the human body. To think about it musically, the body is not a single instrument, hitting a single note. It is a symphony of thousands of different instruments (biochemicals) varying and combining in uncountable ways—all at once, all interactively. Just as individual notes produce a harmony with other notes, so every chemical reaction in a healthy body is functioning in harmony with every other reaction in the body.

It seems clear that to move this entire symphony in a more harmonious direction, it would be most effective to intervene with complex and holistic substances—with supplements that could affect the whole symphony at once. For that, however, you would need some way to know what the formula should be in the first place. Reductionist scientific investigation can't provide that answer. One puzzle is how the ayurvedic vaidyas of ancient times came up with such an effective formula in the first place. It's a puzzle we will consider in Part Three.

In any event, if research can't tease out complex synergistic mechanisms, it can assess overall results. The research evidence on Maharishi Amrit Kalash to date is wide-ranging and impressive. These studies have not only shown marked anti-oxidant effects. They have also shown exactly what one would expect from powerful free radical scavengers—a broad spectrum of specific benefits for specific diseases. Both sets of findings are worth attention in detail.

FREE RADICAL SCAVENGING EFFECTS

Dr. Yukie Niwa was one of the earliest free radical researchers. He has been active in the field for more than 20 years. At his Niwa Institute in Japan he has tested over 500 compounds for their free radical-scavenging effects. Dr. Niwa is an immunologist, and much of his research has focused on the excess inflammation often caused by the immune system.

To begin with, Dr. Niwa and his colleagues conducted chemical analyses of herbs in MAK-4 and MAK-5. These analyses revealed a mixture rich in low-molecular-weight substances that are well-known anti-oxidants, including vitamin C, vitamin E, beta-carotene, polyphenols, bioflavonoids, and riboflavin.[1]

Dr. Niwa then conducted an experiment to document MAK's anti-oxidant effect. His investigation involved the immune system's most rapidly reacting defense force—the neutrophil. As we have seen, once inflammation begins, immune system cells such as neutrophils overproduce free radicals and other ROS, causing extensive damage to healthy cells in the vicinity. Chemicals released by damaged cells encourage rapid transit by neutrophils and other immune cells to the inflammation site, quickly worsening the damage.

Dr. Niwa's study showed that, in the presence of MAK, neutrophil chemotaxis slowed down significantly. In addition, the multiplication of lymphocytes in their most aggressive form (blastogenesis) was also tempered. He also identified the specific reason why MAK-4 and MAK-5 had this tempering effect on the mechanism of inflammation. Both of them markedly scavenged the neutrophil leakage of superoxide, hydrogen peroxide, and the hydroxy radical.[2] According to Dr. Niwa, in fact, MAK scavenged free radicals more effectively than any substance he had tested previously.[3]

Dr. Jeremy Fields and his colleagues at the University of Loyola Medical School in Chicago followed up on Dr. Niwa's work. They focused on superoxide since it is the "master radical"—the first produced and the precursor of both hydrogen peroxide and the hydroxy radical. Fields' group compared MAK with SOD, the enzyme designed specifically to scavenge superoxide. Human immune system cells (neutrophils) were stimulated to create superoxide, as if to kill an invader. MAK and SOD were used to scavenge the superoxide.

The results showed that both MAK and SOD, separately, were able to completely scavenge the superoxide molecules. This was not a surprising finding, after Dr. Niwa's work. The surprise was that MAK proved as every bit as potent as SOD, milligram for milligram. Here was an anti-oxidant that tested to be as powerful as one of the body's tireless enzymes. Because MAK has so many components, Dr. Fields and his colleagues conducted tests to make sure that, in defusing the superoxide, MAK had not damaged the neutrophils themselves. Results showed the neutrophils still healthy and functioning normally.[4]

The implications were significant. First, it indicated that MAK can reduce the random damage caused by neutrophils as they fight invaders. Second, if MAK scavenged superoxide as effectively as the body's own enzyme (SOD), its anti-free radical effectiveness clearly deserved serious attention.

Further experiments reaffirmed MAK's ability to scavenge superoxide.[5] Also, a separate study by Dr. Chandradhar Dwivedi and co-workers at the South Dakota State University showed that MAK-4 and MAK-5 were able to scavenge other dangerous molecules—lipid peroxides.[6]

ONE THOUSAND TIMES MORE EFFECTIVE

At this stage, a number of us at The Ohio State University College of Medicine designed and executed another systematic test of MAK. It had become clear that MAK could stop free radicals. We wanted to know how well.

We decided to do a direct comparison of MAK-4 and -5 with three individual anti-oxidants—vitamin C, vitamin E, and the well-researched drug probucol. We wanted to use quantitative measures to assess the dimensions of this apparent anti-oxidant breakthrough.

We decided to run our test on yet a third damaging molecule—low density lipoprotein (LDL) which had been oxidatively damaged by free radical attack. As we have seen, LDL is known as the "bad" cholesterol. Its poor reputation is not due to its natural state, which is benign, but to its transformed state, after free radical attack. Oxidized LDL (LDL-ox) is itself a particularly damaging free radical. Chapter Three detailed how LDL-ox is central to the process that scars, thickens, and stiffens arterial walls—narrowing the artery passageway and attracting platelets which can aggregate into clots and block the artery entirely. The research indicated that if LDL-ox can be scavenged effectively, cardiovascular disease could be markedly reduced.

For our experiments, we used LDL isolated from human blood samples. To begin a free radical chain reaction, we added copper ions. Copper, like iron, catalyzes a reaction that attacks the double bond in LDL and steals an electron, leaving the LDL altered and radicalized. Once the reaction has begun, it spreads from molecule to molecule of the LDL in a self-perpetuating cascade, as each crippled molecule cripples another.

Because we wanted definitive results, our research design was detailed. One group of tests was run over two periods of time, six hours and 24 hours, after which the incubation mixtures were frozen to stop the reactions. In a different series of tests, the herbal food supplements, vitamins C and E, and probucol were added individually to test tubes containing LDL and copper ions. These substances were also added to test tubes containing LDL without the copper ions. The various substances were added to the test tubes at 0 hours, after 1.5 hours and after 3.5 hours; the incubation of the tubes was continued for a total time of 24 hours. As an experimental control, a parallel set of tubes was run which did not contain the anti-oxidant substances.

Since MAK-4 is a thick paste and MAK-5 a tablet, aqueous and alcoholic extracts were made by dissolving the two supplements in an aqueous solution and an alcoholic solution.

Though the previous studies had given us reason to expect significant findings, the results surprised us nonetheless. As expected, vitamins C and E, probucol, and MAK all prevented the radicalization of LDL if added at time zero. All stopped the ongoing free radical chain reactions if added after 1.5 or 3.5 hours. But the difference in potency was startling. Weight for weight, the aqueous extracts of MAK were several hundred times more potent than vitamins C and E and probucol. The alcoholic extracts were even stronger—at least 1000 times more potent.

In the same study we also tested two other herbal formulas from Maharishi Ayur-Ved. MA-631 is described as similar in purpose to the Maharishi Amrit Kalash formulas. Maharishi Coffee Substitute is an herbal beverage. Each scavenged

LDL-ox radicals with a relative effectiveness that was close to that of MAK.[7]

ASSESSING THE BREAKTHROUGH

I must tell you it is not common to obtain results as potentially significant as these all at once. The scientific process ordinarily moves forward step by step. New discoveries are usually small extensions of previous ones, and the sudden, spectacular leap is extremely rare. Scientific progress, moreover, is often two steps forward and one step back; apparent discoveries from one study frequently disappear in the light of another. For these reasons, people who have made a career of laboratory investigation tend to be quite cautious. Their years in the profession train them to adopt a skeptical stance.

Despite this background, I found it hard to maintain a business-as-usual demeanor in the face of these findings. In the first place, they indicated that there is now an effective means to protect LDL against free radical attack. If this is true, it means there are natural food supplements that can help keep our arteries clear and work adjunctively to prevent a high percentage of heart disease, stroke, and generalized oxygen starvation throughout the body.

In the second place, the results showed that Maharishi Amrit Kalash is an anti-oxidant of unprecedented potency. Vitamin C, vitamin E, and probucol are all well-researched and each has demonstrated the ability to scavenge free radicals and improve specific conditions. To find an anti-oxidant that is literally one thousand times more effective than any of these is to stretch the limits of a researcher's imagination.

Moreover, these findings are consistent with a large body of related research. As this book goes to press, nearly forty studies have been done on MAK worldwide, research conducted by at least fifty investigators representing a broad range of universities and independent research institutions. In these studies, moreover, the findings have painted a consistent picture.

If Maharishi Amrit Kalash is the most effective free radical scavenger, it should enhance health in a significant way. The worldwide research has indicated that this is true. Laboratory and animal studies and human trials have given evidence that MAK's anti-oxidant effects translate into specific benefits for specific diseases. The details give a picture of the possibilities available from synergistic free radical management.

ENHANCING IMMUNITY

A sound immune system is vital to continued health. For this reason, a number of MAK studies have focused on immune functioning. The results have shown that:

1. MAK increases the responsiveness of the immune system.

2. MAK decreases the collateral damage often done by overzealous immune cells.

Both results can be understood in terms of reduced free radical damage.

Researchers at the Indiana University School of Medicine collaborated with others at the University of Kansas and myself to conduct a study on the immune system in laboratory animals. One group of animals received MAK-5 in their diet for 20 days, a second group did not. After the first ten days, the animals were exposed to ovalbumin, an antigen (foreign substance) that challenges the immune system.

The spleen is the generation site for fast-reacting immune system cells (lymphocytes). When spleen cells were challenged with ovalbumin under laboratory conditions, the cells from MAK-fed animals produced two to three times as many lymphocytes as the control animals.[8] This capacity for increased lymphocyte generation persisted for 15 days after MAK was removed from the diet. This increased lymphocyte response was seen only when the lymphocytes were chemically challenged. When they were not challenged, normal proliferation was maintained. This suggests that MAK does not change the normal behavior of lymphocytes, but prepares them for heightened response when they are needed.

Dr. Niwa's study (discussed earlier) demonstrated that this increased responsiveness is kept under control. His double finding—that MAK scavenges free radicals while it also slows the chemotactic attraction of neutrophils—indicated that a more responsive immune system was not going to be a more destructive one.[9]

The tempering effect of MAK-5 on the immune system was also indicated in a study on humans by Dr. Jay Glaser, Medical Director of the Maharishi Ayur-Ved Health Center in Lancaster, Massachusetts. Many common allergic reactions are caused by excessive immune system response. White blood cells react to, say, a particle of pollen as if it were a deadly invading bacteria. The needless damage sown by these overeager defenders results in inflammation of the nasal passages (hay fever) or the lungs (asthma). To test the effectiveness of MAK-5 on this type of immune system overreaction, Dr. Glaser randomly assigned subjects to two groups. One group received Maharishi Amrit Kalash-5. The other group received a placebo pill. Over the next four weeks, a peak allergy season, the group receiving MAK-5 showed significantly fewer allergic symptoms.[10]

Controlling free radical effects on the immune system: MAK's effectiveness against free radicals can reasonably explain both the increased responsiveness of the immune system and the increased control of its tendency to overreact. Since immune system cells are playing with fire, they are uniquely subject to damage. When oxy radicals and ROS released by immune cells damage their own membranes, their functioning is compromised. Cell receptors are crippled,[11] reducing the responsiveness of each cell and the immune system as a whole to the body's wide variety of floating chemical messengers.[12]

Loss of membrane fluidity and destruction of protein machinery embedded in the cell membrane also cause decreased ability of the immune cells to respond to a challenge.[13] Thus, if free radical damage can be significantly controlled, increased responsiveness by the immune system should come about as a natural result.

Free radicals also cause the immune system to spiral out of control. In the inflammatory response, oxy radicals and ROS overreact, and the damage feeds on itself by attracting more and more hyper-excited inflammatory cells into the fray. Anti-oxidants can temper this tendency to self-inflicted damage by rapidly scavenging the excess free radicals released by neutrophils and other cells. The neutrophils, macrophages, and other immune cells can ingest and destroy toxic invaders without causing as much damage to their surroundings—and without attracting an excessive number of their cohorts.

The initial laboratory tests on MAK indicate the presence of both effects. The immune system becomes more responsive and more controlled at the same time. This shows promise for the control of both external (infectious) and internal (degenerative and inflammatory) disease. With the rich variety of molecules in MAK, there may be other mechanisms also involved—including mind-body effects mediated through the limbic system in the brain (see discussion of psychoneuroimmunology below). But MAK's free radical-fighting capabilities go a long way toward explaining these encouraging immune system findings.

CANCER PREVENTION AND REGRESSION

Cancer has been another major area of MAK research. Since cancer is intimately tied to free radical damage, it is no surprise to find that MAK has marked *anti-neoplastic* (anti-cancer) properties.

Prevention and regression of breast carcinoma: The first cancer studies were on breast carcinoma, carried out as a joint project in laboratories at The Ohio State University College of Medicine and Dr. Dwivedi's lab at South Dakota State University. As we have seen, carcinogenesis is ordinarily a two-step process: (1) an apparently irreversible initiation stage, when alterations occur in the DNA of one or more cells, and (2) a promotion stage, in which the population of initiated cells expands. In our first experiment, laboratory animals were fed a diet supplemented with 0.2% MAK-5. They were also exposed to a potent chemical inducer of breast cancer: 7,12 dimethylbenz(a)anthracene (DMBA). An "initiation phase" group of animals received MAK-5 for one week before and one week after DMBA was administered. A "promotion phase" group was given MAK-5 continuously, beginning one week after DMBA was administered. A third combined group was given MAK-5 throughout the experiment.

After 18 weeks, only 25% of the animals receiving MAK-5 during the promotion phase showed tumors, as compared to 67% of animals in the control group. However, in this study with MAK-5, there did not appear to be comparable protection during the initiation phase.[14]

A second experiment with the same design used a diet supplemented with 6% MAK-4. The effects were far more striking. The animals on MAK-4 suffered 60% fewer tumors in the initiation stage and 88% fewer in the promotion phase as compared to control animals.

In addition, in both studies, control animals who had already developed fully-formed tumors were given the MAK diet. In 60% of these animals in both studies, the tumors shrank significantly. In roughly half of those who experienced this tumor regression, the tumor disappeared completely. The animals who experienced this tumor regression were those who initially had tumors under a certain size. Animals with tumors over this size did not improve.[15]

Regression of aggressive lung cancer: Another important study was carried out on lung cancer by Dr. Vimal Patel at Indiana University in collaboration with myself and others. Dr. Patel deliberately chose a challenging type of cancer, Lewis lung carcinoma. This is known to be a cancer which aggressively metastasizes—spreading rapidly to other organs of the body. Rapidly metastasizing cancer is ordinarily the most life-threatening type. This study began with animals who already had Lewis lung carcinoma. MAK-4 was added to their diet, with dramatic results. In 65% of the animals the total number of metastatic nodules decreased, and in 45% the size of the individual nodules also decreased. Once again, a particular cancer condition was actually being reversed.[16]

Increased survival: Dr. Brian Johnston and his colleagues at SRI International (formerly the Stanford Research Institute) studied the effect of MAK on skin tumors. Rather than measure effects on specific tumors, they measured for the most important effect—increased survival. Animals with DMBA-induced papilloma were fed MAK-5 in their diet. The survival rate for MAK-fed animals was 75%, as compared to 31% in the control group.[17]

Prevention of cell transformation: In research supported by the National Cancer Institute (NCI), Julia T. Arnold, with colleagues at NCI (Maryland) and ManTech Environmental Technology, Inc. (North Carolina), studied the anti-cancer effects of MAK with two standardized and frequently-used tests. With one of the tests, MAK inhibited tumor cell growth by up to 50%. With the second test, it inhibited transformation of normal cells to cancer cells by 27–53%. This was the first study to specifically show that MAK could prevent healthy cells from being transformed into cancerous ones.[18]

Transformation of cancer cells to normal cells: The most striking cancer study showed the reverse process— cancerous cells being transformed back into apparently healthy, normal cells—one of the rarest types of reports in the research literature on cancer. It is often said that the initiation stage—damaging alteration to the DNA—is irreversible. This study challenged that supposition. The work was done by Dr. Kedar Prasad, Director of the Center for Vitamin and Cancer Research at the Health Sciences Center, University of Colorado. He did his study on tissue culture cells of neuroblastoma, an aggressive form of neurological cancer most often found in children that is considered extremely difficult to treat. Conventional therapies are known to create severe side effects.

Typical nerve cells are by far the largest cells in the body, with large central bodies and branching dendrites and axons (long, finger-like projections) which can be several feet long. Malignant neuroblastoma cells usually lose much of this nerve cell-style differentiation. They shrink, become circular, and lose the long projections. Once they have reverted to this small, non-specific (undifferentiated) form, they begin to multiply uncontrollably. Dr. Prasad found that MAK-5 reverses this process. Exposed to MAK-5, approximately 75% of the malignant cells appeared to differentiate again—developing the large cell body and dendrites—and to stop their rampant growth.[19] Their biochemical functioning also appeared to return to normal; they produced enzymes that healthy cells usually produce. Only a few agents had previously been reported which cause cancer cells to revert to this normal-like state—and most of them are highly toxic.

Further scientific studies on cancer are now underway, but the reports already available have indicated that taking Maharishi Amrit Kalash as an herbal supplement may help adjunctively to prevent, reverse, and in some cases even eradicate certain cancer conditions. The neuroblastoma study, moreover, makes it seem likely that at least some of the anticancer effects of MAK are due to more than free radical scavenging. For a cell to assume its former, healthy state, the

DNA within the cell must have been reset. Free radicals damage DNA. Anti-oxidants by themselves simply stop the damage. Somewhere within the mystery of the MAK constituents apparently lies the capacity to help reset DNA (see Chapter Eight for a discussion of this point).

REDUCING CARDIOVASCULAR RISK FACTORS

If MAK controls free radicals, it should also produce notable effects on cardiovascular disease. No single benefit could produce a greater improvement in all-around health. As we have seen, atherosclerosis contributes to heart attacks, strokes, and to generalized oxygen and nutrient starvation in tissues and organs everywhere in the body.

At the beginning of this chapter we saw that Maharishi Amrit Kalash has one potent effect that should markedly inhibit the development of atherosclerosis. MAK strongly protects low density lipoprotein (LDL) from free radical attack.[20] Two more studies conducted in our laboratories at Ohio State have shown that MAK can inhibit atherosclerosis in another important way—by inhibiting blood clots due to the aggregation of platelets in the bloodstream.

It's important for platelets to promote blood clotting at the site of serious injury. But an excessive tendency to aggregate into clots can mean that platelets pile up inside blood vessels—at sites of minor cell membrane damage and deposits of fatty streaks. This tendency toward excessive aggregation can be induced by four factors in the body:

1. Catecholamines, such as epinephrine and norepinephrine, which are increased during stress.

2. Collagen, which is exposed when cells lining the vascular walls are injured.

3. Arachidonic acid, which is released by membranes of injured cells.

4. ADP (adenosine diphosphate), which is released from injured red blood cells and platelets.

This chemical pattern means that if stressful living is combined with the type of damage free radicals typically do to blood vessels and bloodstream components, the conditions are perfect for development of dangerous clotting.

In our first study, we obtained blood plasma from normal, healthy adults. Platelet-rich plasma was aliquotted into test tubes. All four inducers of platelet aggregation—epinephrine, collagen, arachidonic acid, and ADP—were tested. When an extract of MAK-5 was added to the plasma, there was a marked inhibition of platelet aggregation in every case.[21] We also tested the effects on whole blood. In this case we used only collagen and ADP, and again MAK-5 potently inhibited platelet aggregation.

Aspirin has become famous for producing such a reduction in platelet aggregation and is now recommended for patients who have already suffered a heart attack. But aspirin has side effects in the gastrointestinal tract and has been linked to an increase in brain hemorrhaging. Aspirin also has no effect on the aggregation caused by ADP. In fact, no previous study has identified a single substance which inhibits aggregation caused by all four of these inducers—and no significant side effects from MAK have been reported (see below).

Reduced cardiovascular risk factors in living animals: It is one thing to get such results in the laboratory. It is also important to see if the benefits carry over into living animals. For a thorough study of cardiovascular risk factors, we tested for overall cholesterol, lipid peroxidation, and platelet aggregation. We fed two groups of six animals a high cholesterol diet. The experimental group was given 0.4% MAK-4 in the diet. After seven weeks, the experiment was concluded and the assays performed.

Overall, the basic cholesterol levels of the MAK animals were one-third less than the controls. In the MAK group, moreover, lipid peroxide levels in the blood (a measure of free radical damage) were nearly two-thirds less than the controls. Finally, in blood from the MAK animals, platelet aggregation induced by collagen was 46% less, and aggregation induced by ADP 82% less. MAK had substantially reduced every risk factor for cardiovascular disease tested in the experiment.[22]

REDUCED CHEMICAL TOXICITY

Even to this point, the research on Maharishi Amrit Kalash must be termed encouraging. MAK is an herbal food, not a drug, yet it has a unique nutritional effectiveness against free radicals, helps work powerfully against risk-factors for heart disease and certain cancer conditions, and helps stimulate and balance particular aspects of the immune system. It is startling to find such wide-ranging effects from an herbal food for dietary use which is employed only as a nutritional addition to the everyday diet.

Yet the research has also identified other significant benefits of MAK. In modern society we have seen that many chemicals have become a major cause of illness and death. This is true of both medications and occupational exposure. Much of the damage caused by these chemicals is due to free radical mechanisms. Exploratory studies have shown that MAK may have a significant role to play in this sphere as well.

Detoxifying adriamycin: For many cancers, adriamycin is a particularly effective medication. Adriamycin works by creating free radicals which destroy the DNA of cancer cells. However, these free radicals damage healthy cells as well. The danger is especially great in the heart, where cells have high levels of oxygen due to their incessant muscular activity.

In collaboration with Dr. Dwivedi at South Dakota State University, we designed a dual experiment to investigate whether MAK, used in conjunction with adriamycin, could reduce the drug's toxic side effects. First, in a laboratory test, we checked to see if MAK could inhibit adriamycin's production of free radicals. Liver microsomes were incubated with a biochemical system that stimulates free radicals. In some cases, adriamycin was added to the system. Alcoholic and aqueous extracts of MAK-4 and MAK-5 were then added as well.

The first results showed that, even in an already efficient biochemical system for creating free radicals, adriamycin increased the production of free radicals by 50%. Second, MAK again proved highly efficient at reducing free radical levels. The alcoholic extract of MAK-5 and both the alcoholic and aqueous extracts of MAK-4 were significantly effective. Both extracts of MAK-4 reduced lipid peroxidation in the microsomes to essentially zero, even in the face of the added free radical load created by adriamycin.[23]

An additional test was conducted on animals that were given adriamycin. One group was fed a standard diet. The other groups received either MAK-4 or MAK-5. At the end of four weeks, the mortality (death rate) among the control group was 60%. The MAK-5 group had a mortality rate one-third lower and the MAK-4 group a mortality rate two-thirds lower. The results of these two experiments indicate that MAK, especially in this case MAK-4, provides substantial protection against the dangerous side effects of a lethal drug.[24]

Protection against toluene: Dr. Stephen Bondy at the University of California, Irvine, has tested MAK against toxic effects of toluene, a hazardous industrial solvent. More than two million American workers are exposed to the dangers of toluene every day—dangers due to toluene's ability to rapidly create free radicals. First, Dr. Bondy's laboratory tests showed that MAK effectively scavenged free radicals created by toluene. Next, a study was done on laboratory animals. Animals were first given MAK-5 for two days, then exposed to toluene. Examinations revealed a significant reduction of free radical formation in the MAK-5 group as compared to the control group.[25]

ANTI-AGING EFFECTS

One of the most intriguing questions in free radical research is whether effective free radical control can slow the aging process and extend life. Three preliminary studies on MAK have been encouraging.

Dr. Jeremy Fields' team at the University of Loyola conducted two of these experiments. In the first test, MAK was fed as a dietary supplement to laboratory mice starting at the age of 18 months (roughly 50–60 years of age in human terms). Even starting at this relatively advanced age, 80% of the MAK group survived to 23 months of age compared to only 48% survival for the control group. To check for effects throughout a life span, Dr. Fields turned to an experimental standby—the fruit fly. Fruit flies thrive and breed well in the laboratory, but their natural life span is only weeks long, allowing complete experiments in a short period of time. In this case, fruit flies fed MAK from birth lived 70% longer than controls.[26]

A provocative human test has also been conducted by Dr. Paul Gelderloos and his associates at Maharishi International University (MIU) in Fairfield, Iowa. (Founded by Maharishi Mahesh Yogi, MIU combines a traditional academic education with twice daily practice of Transcendental Meditation. MIU has been accredited through the Ph.D. level and scientific research there has been frequently supported by grants from various branches of the National Institutes for Health, as well as the National Science Foundation and other federal and private sources.)

Dr. Gelderloos reasoned that if MAK has a positive effect on aging, this should show up in measurements of age-related functioning. He chose a complex test combining both visual acuity and mental processing—to assess complex functioning of the nervous system. The test involves cards which have an array of letters laid out regularly in a grid. The grid contains 110 "X's" and one "V". The lone V tends to get lost in the sea of X's. The X's act as distractions (known as *noise*), attracting attention away from the target stimulus. Previous research on such tests had shown that the ability to quickly pick out the V worsens markedly with age[27]—due partly to physical deterioration (reduced retinal metabolism[28]) and partly to an age-related deficit in information processing.[29]

Dr. Gelderloos used a stringent research design. He first pair-matched 48 men for similar age and education, then randomly assigned one from each pair to one of two groups. One of the groups was given MAK-5, the second a placebo tablet manufactured to closely mimic the MAK tablet. Before the men started taking the tablets, they were given the visual test—with many variations of the X's and V, each variation flashed on the screen for about three-tenths of a second. They were asked to locate the V and mark its location on sheets they were provided. They were tested again after taking the tablets twice a day for three weeks, and again after six weeks. The experimenters and the people who scored the tests were not told which men were taking MAK and which the placebo.

The results supported the hypothesis. First, performance on the test, both for the MAK and placebo group, was strongly correlated with age. The younger men consistently scored the highest. Second, the group which took MAK improved significantly more than the placebo group in all age ranges after both three and six weeks.[30]

Such statistically significant improvement in a matter of weeks would be difficult to explain if it were not for the free radical paradigm. Long-range testing is still needed, but Dr. Gelderloos' work has demonstrated that MAK's unparalleled free-radical scavenging ability can apparently rejuvenate cell functioning—thus improving a complex physical/mental process and producing more youthful functioning.

Re-differentiation and rejuvenation: We have discussed the dysdifferentiation theory of Dr. Richard Cutler from the National Institute of Aging—the idea that cells "forget" what specific type they are supposed to be. They regress (dysdifferentiate) to a generic and generally useless form. Dr. Cutler speculates that free radical damage to the DNA causes this dysdifferentiation.

This theory has relevance to the MAK research. Dr. Cutler has expressed hope that anti-oxidants might slow the rate of dysdifferentiation. The study by Dr. Prasad on neuroblastoma cells (mentioned above) has shown something even better. In certain circumstances, at least, loss of differentiation can actually be reversed.

In Dr. Prasad's study, cancer cells incubated with MAK returned to an apparently normal style of functioning. His study also showed that as long as the newly re-differentiated cells continued to be cultured with MAK, they maintained their healthy, normal status. MAK appeared to help maintain their differentiation.[31] This implies at least the possibility that regular use of MAK could help to maintain proper differentiation of bodily cells. If such differentiation continued in the most important glands of the body, which are Dr. Cutler's focus, then proper hormone levels would be maintained in the physiology as a whole. The aging process could be significantly retarded. It's an intriguing hypothesis that warrants further testing.

MIND AND BODY

Based on the ancient ayurvedic descriptions, we might expect that Maharishi Amrit Kalash would have effects beyond its potent free radical scavenging. Specifically, in the ayurvedic tradition, herbal supplements such as MAK were said to lead not only to improved physical health, but also to enhanced psychological well-being. From one perspective, this is only logical. Physical health and psychological health go hand in hand.

Such mind-body connections are a leading topic in medical research. Modern medicine has recently begun to find objective evidence to support what most doctors once knew from their own practice: feeling good can make you well. It is commonplace experience that stress and tension, anxiety and fear, sadness and disappointment can all lead to illness. This simple observation was once the basis of the family physician's warm and reassuring bedside manner. Every good doctor knew that if patients felt comforted and encouraged, they would do better. Today, however, family doctors are a disappearing species, and fear of a malpractice suit has led doctors to reverse their style; they tell their patients every conceivable catastrophe their symptoms might lead to—lest they be accused of incompetence.

Research in the last decade makes the old bedside manner look like the better medicine. It has been well established that stress affects mental functioning, which in turn affects physiological functioning[32]—largely because stress creates free radicals in abundance. In addition, severe mental depression has been shown to result in suppression or total loss of immune system functioning.[33] On the other hand, a positive mental state correlates with increased survival time for some patients with AIDS and cancer.[34]

Investigators have begun to explain these relationships. They are identifying a rich physiological network connecting mind and body. They have begun to identify an objective basis of mind-body medicine.

FEELINGS TO MOLECULES:
THE LIMBIC CONNECTION

The heart of this network is called the *limbic system*—the pituitary gland (the body's master gland), which nestles under the hypothalamus (the body's central regulatory switchboard), which is surrounded by the limbic area of the brain (the physiological seat of emotions). In this one small area at the base of the brain, there is a close physiological connection between feelings and the functioning of the body.

The limbic region itself is that part of the brain that correlates with deep emotional states. It surrounds the hypothalamus, which has often been called the "brain's brain." The hypothalamus regulates temperature, thirst, hunger, blood sugar levels, growth, sleeping and waking, and emotions such as anger and happiness. Situated just below the hypothalamus is the pituitary, which emits secretions that control the activity of many other glands in the body. Taken together, this limbic system alters with every alteration in emotions—creating a new mix of molecules which transforms the functioning of the physical body.

Stimuli coming from the limbic region of the brain cause the hypothalamus to release a wide variety of neuropeptides. These neuropeptides, in turn, stimulate specific hormones from the pituitary gland and, thus, specific activity in all endocrine glands, including the thymus and adrenal glands. This new combination of chemical messengers changes the operation and make-up of the body.

Through the action of the limbic system, particular psychological and emotional states take on molecular form. When you watch an action movie, you may begin to feel a nervous stomach and sweaty palms. Specific chemical messengers have been released. The body has been changed by what it is seeing on the screen. The emotions raised by the movie correlate with activity in the limbic system.

In this sense, the body metabolizes the emotional content of every experience it has. Happiness registering in the limbic region stimulates one cascade of chemicals from the hypothalamus and pituitary, with corresponding physiological change everywhere in the body. Sadness creates another cascade, and another physiology. What you feel, you become. Even fleeting moods, altered by fleeting thoughts, change the biochemical output of this system. Different neuropeptides and hormones are made. They have different effects throughout the body. The contents of consciousness alter the physiology.

Mind-body shortcut: The hypothalamus can also communicate with the body directly. Neuropeptides produced by the hypothalamus are not received by the pituitary alone. In fact, they can be received by receptors on cells throughout the body. An action movie can create a nervous stomach because the digestive tract has receptors for stress-response neuropeptides created in the hypothalamus.

Most significantly, these receptors have been found on immune system lymphocytes all over the body.[35] Apparently, lymphocytes can tune in to the molecular messages created by thoughts and feelings. On the other hand, chemicals created by the lymphocytes, such as interleukins, have receptors in the hypothalamic region of the brain. Thus, chemical messages from the immune system can modulate nervous system functioning and mental states.[36] So there is a two-way communication network between the brain and the immune system. A growing body of data also suggests that neurotransmitters produced by the autonomic nervous system can communicate directly with the immune system and modify its functioning.

The mind, nervous system, and immune system are thus tied together in a network that was discovered as long as a decade ago. The connection between moods and health is no longer mysterious. Negative emotions depress the immune system through this psychophysiological connection. A reassuring bedside manner actually creates medicine inside the body—it stimulates the production of neuropeptides that "encourage" the immune cells. These discoveries have led to the new field of psychoneuroimmunology[37] and have produced a solid footing for mind-body medicine. The mind and body connect through molecules.

Mind, body, and MAK: These new findings help to explain how an herbal food supplement—a physical substance—can have psychological effects. The molecular connection between mind and body is beginning to make sense of such integrated effects.

Because of the ancient predictions that MAK would have mental as well as physical benefits, we decided to test its effects both on psychological mood and on biochemical operation in the brain. We began with a much-utilized questionnaire that gauges emotional well-being. When given to people using MAK, the results of this questionnaire showed marked improvements in psychological mood—greater happiness, tranquility, mental clarity, and emotional balance.[38]

Was there any physiological explanation for these changes? To check for a molecular connection, we investigated the interaction of MAK with receptors in the brain known as opioid receptors. Opiate drugs, such as morphine, attach to these receptors. There was much publicity a few years ago when researchers discovered that the body has natural opioids, endorphins and enkephalins, that also lock onto these receptors. These can act as natural painkillers, and they also produce positive emotions, create a more relaxed and stable style of operation in the autonomic nervous system, and modify the functioning of the immune system.

Our tests showed that MAK did in fact interact with these receptors. One or more of the components in MAK was docking in the same place the natural opioids attach. This suggests that MAK could stimulate the same response among brain cells—producing more positive emotions, and a calming effect on the nervous system, while also influencing the immune system.[39]

Fighting depression: A study done at MIU in Fairfield, Iowa, further demonstrated MAK's mind-body role. Imipramine is one of the major prescription drugs given for depression. It binds strongly with a receptor in brain cells that increases the output of serotonin—one of the most thoroughly studied neurotransmitters. Low levels of serotonin correlate with aggression, hostility, and other mental health problems.[40] High levels of serotonin correlate with a comfortable, even exhilarated emotional tone.[41] Imipramine, the serotonin trigger, binds not only to brain cells but also to blood platelets, providing another tie between mind and body.

The research at MIU showed that MAK interacted with the same receptor on blood platelets as imipramine. This suggests that MAK might bind to the same receptor in brain cells, increasing serotonin levels and thus providing a positive effect on both psychological mood and immune system functioning.[42]

Reducing inflammation and pain: A separate study reported that subjects using MAK-5 for three months showed a significant decrease in substance P, another neurotransmitter. Substance P is triggered by pain and is associated with pulmonary and gastrointestinal inflammation. Reduction of substance P thus indicates that MAK may be able to reduce such inflammation and its associated pain.[43]

These studies are encouraging. A fulfilling life depends on both physical and mental health. Put another way, we all seek good health and happiness. There is evidence to show that MAK stimulates both. These studies go beyond the free radical paradigm and indicate that MAK may have effects on consciousness as well as the physiology. It's a topic we will return to in Part Three.

LACK OF SIDE EFFECTS

Our experience with modern medicine has taught us to always look for negative results along with the positive. In the ayurvedic tradition, however, it has long been asserted that Amrit Kalash and other ayurvedic supplements have no significant side effects. The mixture of components is said to increase the potency, while also balancing biochemical influences and thus negating destructive side effects. The research to date has supported this view.

A cross-sectional survey of 659 men and women who had been taking MAK for an average of 22 months reported a wide range of benefits but no significant side effects. In addition, a pilot study of 126 subjects using MAK and many other modalities of Maharishi Ayur-Ved showed only five per cent with even minor side effects.[44] The most common were skin rash and gastrointestinal disturbance—and these responded to reduced dosage.

To rule out toxicity more explicitly, a blood examination was carried out on 84 subjects who had been using MAK for at least six months. Standard tests of biochemical, hematological, and liver enzyme parameters revealed no toxic effects.[45] A separate study performed the same blood tests on nine subjects tested before and after taking MAK-5 for three months. Again, the blood samples were normal and no toxic effects were found.[46]

TIPPING THE SCALES

Maharishi Amrit Kalash may challenge the preconceptions of modern science. It may be a sumptuously non-reductive melange of thousands of different molecules. But it has passed the most important of all scientific tests. It produces results.

In fact, the studies indicate that it works much more effectively than the best-known anti-oxidants—and that it fights a wide range of diseases.

MAK includes natural anti-oxidants—vitamins, beta-carotene, polyphenols, and bioflavonoids—in high concentration. It also includes a myriad of substances not yet isolated and examined in the laboratory. Modern medicine leans toward isolated active ingredients, usually produced artificially. But ayurvedic vaidyas maintain that complex herbal mixtures of properly chosen and prepared ingredients are much more effective. They maintain that the natural synergism not only increases the mixture's potency, but also works to mitigate any side effects caused by individual components.

In the case of free radicals, and the wide-ranging damage free radicals cause, the research on Maharishi Amrit Kalash apparently upholds the ayurvedic view. To the extent these studies are accurate, therefore, they not only define a breakthrough for prevention and treatment of disease. They also amount to a breakthrough in medical theory itself. Confronted with the most basic cause of illness and aging yet discovered by modern science, scientists have shown that isolated active ingredients—magic bullets—do not work nearly as well as the rich natural formulations of ayurveda. A deeper understanding of the cause of disease has led to a clear demonstration of the benefits produced by natural synergism.

Thus, the very effectiveness of Maharishi Amrit Kalash raises intriguing questions about the health care theory that stands behind it. It has been shown that MAK can help to tip the scales against free radicals—thus reducing the constant load of oxidative stress in the body and improving physical health in many measurable ways. With such fundamental effects on health, it seems likely that these herbal formulations did not appear accidentally—but are rather the result of a comprehensive theory of health and health care.

Before we move on to such questions, however, there is another body of research that is equally promising. It is one thing to control free radicals after they have been generated.

It is quite another thing—and arguably even more significant—to prevent their creation in the first place.

We have seen that chronic stress results in constant free radical generation. This means that effective stress management should slow the creation of excess free radicals—and significantly improve physical health. It is time to look at the evidence showing you can fight free radicals in a completely different way—while sitting in a chair with your eyes closed.

Notes

1. Sharma HM, et al, *Pharmacol Biochem Behav* 35(1990): 767-73

2. Niwa Y, *Indian J Clin Prac* 1(1991): 23-7

3. Niwa Y, personal communication (1989)

4. Fields JZ, et al, *Pharmacologist* 32(1990): A155 (Abstract)

5. Tomlinson PF Jr., Wallace RK, *J Fed Am Soc Exper Biol* 5(1991): A1284 (Abstract)

6. Dwivedi C, et al, *Pharmacol Biochem Behav* 39(1991): 649-52

7. Sharma HM, et al, *Pharmacol Biochem Behav* 43(1992): 1175-82

8. Dileepan KN, et al, *Biochem Arch* 6(1990): 267-74

9. Niwa, *Indian* (see note 1)

10. Glaser JL, et al, *Proc Am Assoc Ayurvedic Med* 7(1991): 6

11. Bendich A, "Antioxidant Nutrients and Immune Functions" in *Antioxidant Nutrients and Immune Functions*, Bendich A, et al, eds. (Plenum Press, New York, 1990), pp. 1-12

12. Erickson KL, et al, *Lipids* 18(1983): 468-474

13. Fountain MW, Schultz RD, *Mol Immunol* 19(1982): 59-64

14. Sharma HM, et al, *Jour Res Edu Ind Med* 10(3)(1991): 1-8; Sharma HM, et al, *American Physiological Society and the American Society for Pharmacology and Experimental Therapeutics* (1988): A121 (Abstracts)

15. Ibid; Sharma HM, et al, *Pharmacol Biochem Behav* 35(1990): 767-73

16. Patel VK, et al, *Nutr Res* 12(1992): 667-76

17. Johnston BH, et al, *Pharmacologist* 3(1991): 39 (Abstract)

18. Arnold JT, et al, *Proc Am Assoc Cancer Res* 32(1991): 128 (Abstract)

19. Prasad KN, et al, *Neuropharmacology* 31(1992): 599-607

20. Sharma, *Pharmacol* (see note 7)

21. Sharma HM, et al, *Clin Ter Cardiovasc* 8(1989): 227-30

22. Panganamala RV, Sharma HM, *International Atherosclerosis Society, 9th Int'l Sympos Atheroscler* (Rosemont, IL,USA, Oct. 6-11, 1991) (Abstract)

23. Engineer FN, et al, *Biochem Arch* 8(1992): 267-72

24. Ibid

25. Bondy S, et al, *Biochem Arch* (1993)(in press)

26. Fields JZ, et al, *J Fed Am Soc Exper Biol* 5(1991): A1735 (Abstract)

27. Gilmore GC, et al, *J Gerontol* 40(1985): 586-92; Sekuler R, Ball K, *J Optic Soc Am* (section A) 3(1986): 864-7

28. Wolf E, *Highw Res Record* 167(1967): 1-7

29. Plude DJ, Hoyer WJ, "Attention and Performance: Identifying and Localizing Age Deficits" in *Aging and Performance*, Charness N, ed. (Wiley, London, 1985), pp. 47-99

30. Gelderloos P, et al, *Int J Psychosomat* 37(1990): 25-9

31. Prasad, *Neuropharmacol* (see note 19)

32. Plotnikoff N, et al, *Stress and Immunity* (CRC Press, Boca Raton, 1991)

33. Hillhouse JE, et al, "Stress-associated Modulation of the Immune Response in Humans," Ibid, pp. 3-27

34. Derogatis LR, et al, *JAMA* 242(1979): 1504-9; Solomon GF, et al, *Ann NY Acad Sci* 496(1987): 647-55; Solomon G, *Advances* 2(1985): 6-19

35. Faith RE, et al, "Interactions Between the Immune System and the Nervous System" in *Stress and Immunity* (see note 32), pp. 287-303

36. Ibid

37. Ader R, "A Historical Account of Conditioned Immunobiologic Response" in *Psychoneuroimmunology*, Ader R, ed. (Academic Press, New York, 1981)

38. Blasdell KS, et al, *J Fed Am Soc Exper Biol* 5(1991): A1317 (Abstract)

39. Sharma HM, et al, *Jour Res Edu Ind Med* 10(1)(1991): 1-8

40. Higley JD, et al, *Arch Gen Psychiatry* 49(1992): 436-41; Kruesi MJP, et al, *Arch Gen Psychiatry* 49(1992): 429-35

41. Charney DS, et al, *Psychopharmacol* 77(1982): 217-22

42. Hauser T, et al, *Society for Neuroscience, 18th Annual Meeting* 14(1988): 244 (Abstract)

43. Sharma, *Jour* (see note 39)

44. Janssen GWHM, *Ned Tijdschr Geneeskd* 5(1989): 56-94

45. Blasdell, *J Fed* (see note 38)

46. Sharma, *Jour* (see note 39)

CHAPTER SIX

Stopping Free Radicals Before They Start

Stress is one of America's leading causes of disease and death. Chronic stress leads to mental frustration, anxiety, and ultimately depression. Chronic stress also breaks out physically as headaches, allergies, ulcers, and heart disease. Ultimately, stress wears the immune system down, and the body becomes prey to disease. Sooner or later, chronic, untreated stress will make you ill.

In the last chapter, we saw how the physical body metabolizes every experience through the action of the limbic system. Every thought and mood creates its own molecules—its own biochemical reality. Under the constant experience of stress, the hypothalamus releases neuropeptides that keep the body chronically excited. Due to the chemical messages from the hypothalamus, the pituitary stimulates the adrenal glands to release a constant barrage of stress hormones—cortisol, epinephrine, norepinephrine, and others. In Chapter Two, we saw how this unleashes a continual free radical bombardment on every cell in the body:

1. Stress hormones stoke the cells' energy furnaces, and excess free radicals are created as an inevitable by-product.

2. Stress hormones trigger chemical reactions that release free radicals.

3. Some stress hormones break down into aldehyde free radicals that tie molecules in knots—while epinephrine and others can turn into redox-cycling free radical factories.[1]

Under stress, the free radical balance in the body is constantly tipped in the wrong direction. Systematic damage is the inevitable result.

What's worse, virtually everyone in modern society lives under an increasing load of stress. Some workplaces are more stressful and some less, but anyone who must work for a living suffers from stress. Tensions and pressures of home life can also be stressful, as can the constant shortage of time most people live with. Traffic is stressful. The TV news is stressful. School is stressful. The ever-present danger of crime is stressful. All of this stress is metabolized by the body. We have developed a society that makes us sick.

THE FIRST SCIENTIFIC MEDITATION

In the last chapter we found evidence that the ancient tradition of ayurvedic medicine supplies uniquely effective herbal food supplements to fight free radicals once they are created. In this chapter, we will look at research on another strategy from the Vedic tradition: meditation. In medical terms, this approach is designed to stop free radicals before they start—by reducing stress and tension.

Extensive scientific research on meditation began with the Transcendental Meditation technique taught by Maharishi Mahesh Yogi. Even in the late 1950s, when Maharishi first began his teaching in the West, it was obvious that industrial civilization was dangerous to mental and physical health. What wasn't obvious then is that meditation could help.

Right up until 1970, when the first research on Transcendental Meditation began to appear, few doctors or psychologists had ever considered meditation as a health-creating technology. If meditation was thought about at all, prevailing wisdom said it was mystical and probably, at basis, illusory. The vague notions of meditation then in circulation involved caves and nail beds, arduous concentration and pointless trance. At best, meditation was considered impractical, for dropouts and dreamers eager to forego life in the real world.

During the 1960s, Maharishi became the best-known meditation teacher anywhere in the world. He continually urged a new understanding of meditation. He explained that his Transcendental Meditation technique was not mystical or religious, but a practical technology to increase success in daily life. Correct meditation, he insisted, involves no concentration or mental effort. It is natural and effortless, and easy to learn. It takes only 20 minutes twice a day.

He especially emphasized that there is no need to run away from life's responsibilities. He maintained that everyday distractions cannot prevent anyone from enjoying the deep inner experience of meditation. He described this experience as one of profound inner silence—with the mind wide awake, but perfectly still. With a correct meditation technique, Maharishi said, the human mind will settle down effortlessly to this silent state because, "It's the natural tendency of the mind. Once we give the mind the correct angle it will settle down automatically to more refined levels. . . . This makes the mind more awake. And when our awareness has gained maximum wakefulness, the next step of refinement transcends the field of thinking. We attain a field of 'pure' awareness. The mind is awake within itself, but without a thought."[2]

Such silent inner wakefulness would give the body a completely new experience to metabolize. Instead of metabolizing stress, with self-destructive results, it could metabolize peace and inner contentment. The recent mind-body discoveries centering on the limbic system suggest that this meditative state might recreate the body in ways that could lead to improved physical health.

In the 1960s, however, the limbic system was little understood, and the state of maximum wakefulness or pure awareness was essentially unknown to Western science. To the best of conventional understandings, a person was either awake (aware of the world around him), asleep (without such awareness), or dreaming (aware of an imaginary world). Maharishi was positing a *fourth* state of consciousness (maximum wakefulness but without thoughts—*pure* awareness). The questions posed by this teaching were many. Did such a fourth state really exist? That is, did meditation really do anything? How could you tell? What good did it do? Maharishi maintained that among other things, this deep inner experience dissolves stress and tension, but there was no objective evidence to show he was right.

From the beginning of his teaching, however, Maharishi encouraged scientists to test his ideas through research. It took 13 years, until 1970, before the first study appeared. Physiologist R. Keith Wallace did a series of experiments at UCLA which were published in *Science* magazine, the *American Journal of Physiology*, and *Scientific American*.

The floodgates were open, and the outpouring of research on a subject once considered mystical and unscientific has been remarkable. Scholars wishing to master the field have a challenging task. On all meditation and relaxation techniques put together, one report lists more than 1200 studies to date.[3] On the Transcendental Meditation technique alone, more than 500 studies have been conducted at 210 universities and research centers in 30 countries around the world. The results have been published in more than 100 academic journals, and the collected papers on Transcendental Meditation fill more than 3,500 oversized pages in five volumes.

There are two reasons why Dr. Wallace's first studies on Transcendental Meditation had such impact. First, they made it clear that meditation did, in fact, do something—it produced a state of unique physical relaxation while also producing unusual changes in brain wave patterns. Second, these studies gave birth to the field of stress management, a field still growing today. For the first time, research showed there was a simple way to relieve stress, tension, and anxiety—without recourse to pills.

RELAXING THE BODY

Over the last two decades researchers have investigated this topic thoroughly, and the evolution of their discoveries has been intriguing. Though it might seem that all relaxation is the same, research has shown something quite different. Most relaxation leads to sleepiness and mental dullness. Transcendental Meditation, however, is purported to result in physical relaxation and, simultaneously, mental alertness—a state Dr. Wallace called "restful alertness." Meditation research has matured since 1970, and these points have now been investigated in many published studies.

In the early days of meditation research, there was much focus on the total amount of oxygen being used by the body during meditation. If you relax, in theory, you don't burn as much oxygen. Relaxation seemingly equates with less oxygen consumption. In the first studies on Transcendental Meditation, and on other relaxation and meditation techniques invented by medical investigators, there were reports of lowered overall oxygen consumption.

As the research effort went forward, however, measuring equipment improved and research designs became more stringent. With more rigorous testing, oxygen consumption turned out to be not such a clear-cut marker of the meditation experience. The amount of oxygen consumed during meditation was found to be highly variable—from person to person, and from experiment to experiment. In some controlled studies on Transcendental Meditation, the rate of oxygen consumption dropped significantly more than it does in eyes-closed resting. In other studies, it did not. At the same time, a number of studies reported that heart rate during meditation did not always drop significantly more than in eyes-closed resting either.

At this point, some researchers abandoned their studies. They assumed that if oxygen consumption and heart rate were not reliable measures of meditation, then meditation did not produce significant rest or relaxation. They wrote meditation off and moved on to other topics.

One lab, however, pressed forward with the research. At the University of California (Irvine) Medical Center, Dr. A.F. Wilson, the Chief of Pulmonary Medicine, worked with his colleague, Dr. Ronald Jevning, and others on a series of detailed studies comparing people practicing the Transcendental Meditation technique with others sitting with eyes closed. Dr. Wilson does not meditate himself, but he was intrigued with some highly unusual findings his team made in their early investigations.

One thing they found was that during Transcendental Meditation, metabolism in arm muscles dropped significantly.[4] There was no change in a control group. This indicated that the body's musculature was relaxing. Wilson and Jevning also found that, in blood withdrawn while subjects meditated, red blood cells also showed reduced metabolism. This was a highly unusual finding. Ordinarily, red blood cells don't slow down even during sleep. Floating in the bloodstream, they have no direct connection with the operation of the nervous system. Their metabolism ordinarily remains constant 24 hours a day. Finally, the team found that during Transcendental Meditation, blood flow to the arms and legs, and also to the internal organs, decreased markedly. During ordinary rest, blood flow to the internal organs *increases* (thus encouraging digestion, for example).

Dr. Wilson's team faced two puzzles. First, their precise studies had shown that during Transcendental Meditation there was a clear pattern of physical rest and relaxation —reduced metabolism in muscles and blood cells—even if earlier studies on overall oxygen consumption had been ambiguous. Second, blood flow decreased to extremities and internal organs, but the heart rate did not slow down. Both puzzles came down to one: If the heart is still pumping normally, where does the missing blood go?

The group hypothesized that, during Transcendental Meditation, there must be a significant increase in blood flow to the brain. People who practice Transcendental Meditation report feeling more alert and awake than usual. Maharishi maintains that Transcendental Meditation improves the quality of consciousness. Perhaps increased blood flow to the brain supplies oxygen and nutrients for increased brain cell activity—while, at the same time, keeping the heart rate and overall oxygen consumption relatively normal.

The study was done, and the hypothesis proved correct. There was a marked increase in cerebral blood flow.[5] A completely new pattern of physiological activity had been discovered—overall physiological rest and relaxation combined with an enriched blood supply in the brain.

COMPARATIVE RESEARCH ON MEDITATION

The differences between meditation and normal rest were further investigated in a major comparative study conducted by Dr. Michael Dillbeck and Dr. David Orme-Johnson of the psychology department at Maharishi International University. Dr. Dillbeck has published many key studies on meditation in academic journals, and Dr. Orme-Johnson has published more meditation research than any other scholar in the world. In this study, Dr. Dillbeck and Dr. Orme-Johnson wanted to produce a definitive analysis, a thorough examination that could be repeated by any other scholar.

They began their work with a literature search. They found 31 scientific papers reporting experiments previously conducted at many different universities and research institutions. Each study took measurements on people during Transcendental Meditation and/or on people sitting with eyes closed. Using a standard mathematical procedure called *meta-analysis*, Dr. Dillbeck and Dr. Orme-Johnson produced a statistical comparison. Such a meta-analysis is considered more accurate than an individual study by itself, because it compares data from an extensive group of subjects. Also, a meta-analysis is completely objective; any other researchers can undertake their own literature search and replicate the statistical analysis.

The study showed that on several parameters Transcendental Meditation produced a level of rest much deeper than eyes-closed resting:

1. During Transcendental Meditation the autonomic nervous system settled down and became much more stable than during eyes-closed resting.

2. The rate of respiration during Transcendental Meditation slowed down significantly more than in eyes-closed resting (even though total oxygen consumption was not significantly lower).

3. Compared to the resting control groups, the Transcendental Meditation subjects showed a much larger decrease in plasma lactate—a chemical marker of metabolic activity.[6]

The study concluded that Transcendental Meditation produces a unique pattern of physiological relaxation, clearly deeper than the rest during simple eyes-closed resting.

A FOURTH STATE OF CONSCIOUSNESS

Many researchers feel that the distinctive changes in physiological functioning during Transcendental Meditation support Maharishi's description of a fourth state of consciousness. It is well known that during the three common states of consciousness—waking, sleeping, and dreaming—the body functions in three completely different ways. For every state of consciousness, there is a distinctly different style of physical functioning. Breathing during sleep is slow and heavy. Breathing during dreaming is lighter, and there are sometimes movements of the eyes and limbs.

To many researchers, Transcendental Meditation, viewed in detail, paints a picture of a totally new style of physical functioning. There are many signs of deep relaxation— reduced muscle and red blood cell metabolism, more stable nervous system functioning, and decreases in breath rate and blood lactate. At the same time, blood flow to the brain increases in a highly distinctive way, and—as we will see shortly—there are also distinctive changes in the brain's electrical activity. Overall, this style of physical functioning is completely different from the style seen during waking, sleeping, or dreaming.

Maharishi's assertion that Transcendental Meditation produces a fourth state of consciousness can't be tested directly. Because consciousness is purely subjective, it can't be measured objectively. But you *can* measure the body's physical operation. You can measure breath rate, blood flow, nervous system stability. These outer signs reflect changes deep within the limbic system, and we have seen that changes within the limbic system reflect changes in consciousness. During Transcendental Meditation, such measurements have demonstrated a new, fourth style of functioning. Like paleontologists reconstructing a prehistoric animal from its skeleton, physiologists have inferred a fourth state of consciousness from this fourth style of physical operation.

Is this fourth state useful? Does it produce long-term results? It would be of little help in the fight against free radicals, for instance, if the deep relaxation experienced during meditation lasted only 20 minutes. If high stress levels immediately returned, cranking out free radicals at a rapid rate, meditation would be a temporary escape, but not a solution.

On the other hand, the facts covered in the last chapter indicate that the limbic system can metabolize the deep inner experience of meditation. This peaceful experience should therefore produce a new combination of biochemicals. This could help break the cycle of constant stress—and reset the body to a more stable and relaxed style of functioning.

The meta-analysis conducted by Dr. Dillbeck and Dr. Orme-Johnson addressed this question as well. In all the previously conducted studies being compared, people practicing Transcendental Meditation and/or people sitting with eyes closed were measured *before* the meditation or eyes-closed resting began. In these measurements, people who had been practicing Transcendental Meditation twice a day showed signs of much deeper relaxation—even though they had not meditated for several hours previously. In these "baseline" measurements—taken before the experiment began—the meditators showed lower heart rate, lower respiration rate, lower plasma lactate, and more nervous system stability.[7] Apparently, the regular inner experience of silence and peace had tuned their bodies to a more stable and relaxed style of functioning. In effect, it appeared, their free radical factories had been slowed down.

STRESS MANAGEMENT THROUGH MEDITATION

Since the 1970s, when the research on Transcendental Meditation began to appear, many other meditation and stress management techniques have been invented and scientifically studied. It has often been said that all of these techniques reduce stress with about equal effectiveness. But this is a question that can be, and has been, studied in statistical detail —in an even more thorough meta-analysis. In this exhaustive study, nearly two decades of stress-related studies have been compared statistically, with the results printed in the *Journal of Clinical Psychology*.

The original studies used in this meta-analysis measured emotional anxiety, because the first emotional sign of stress is an increase in anxiety. Constant tension makes people feel uneasy and worried. Because meditation and relaxation techniques are supposed to reduce stress, psychologists have tested their effects on anxiety more than on any other parameter.

Stanford researcher Dr. Kenneth Eppley decided to do a search for such anxiety studies and found more than 100. These studies tested the effectiveness of every well-known meditation or relaxation technique, including Transcendental Meditation, other types of meditation, the much-researched Progressive Muscle Relaxation technique, the relaxation response, and many others. Using the statistical methods of meta-analysis, Dr. Eppley compared all the techniques. The results challenged the common perception that all meditation and relaxation techniques are equally effective. In the results of all the tests together, the Transcendental Meditation technique reduced anxiety more than twice as much as any other technique.[8]

Dr. Eppley had so many studies to work with that he was able to make some important breakdowns in the statistical data. One of the most important of these breakdowns looked at those studies with the best research designs.

In any new field of research, it is typical that the first research studies—called *pilot* studies—are fairly simple tests to see if results are produced and if more research is warranted. These first studies are often done quickly and inexpensively, with less-than-rigorous research designs. For instance, they may be done with only one-time testing (a *cross-sectional* study), rather than pre-post testing with a time lag in between (a *prospective* or *longitudinal* study). They may not have a large number of subjects—which makes the results less definitive. They may not have a control group—which makes it harder to rule out alternative explanations for the findings. If they use a control group, they may not use random assignment to the control group—which means that people can "self-select" into the experimental and control groups, and self-selected subjects may bring biases and predispositions with them. Even with control groups, there may be a large dropout rate among test subjects before the study ends—which can seriously bias the results. For example, if all the most anxious people drop out of the study, leaving only the less anxious people to take the final test, the post-test would show less anxiety even if the meditation technique itself had no effect.

These issues have often been raised with meditation research. In the 1970s, many initial studies on all techniques used less-than-rigorous designs. It is possible to say that positive results from some of these studies might have been due to sloppy design. According to this criticism, researchers who were biased toward a specific meditation or relaxation technique might get the results they wanted if the studies were not rigorous enough.

Dr. Eppley was in a position to answer such questions definitively. First, he analyzed all the results to see which aspects of research design actually made a difference in this body of research. He found two factors most significant—random assignment to control groups and dropout rate (known as *attrition*). From the overall group of more than 100 studies, he then chose only those studies which had both random assignment and low attrition. All these studies had been published in academic journals or conducted as doctoral dissertations under the guidance of academic experts.

The results of this comparison did show that more stringent research design deflated results for most techniques.
With rigorous methodologies, these techniques produced a
reduction of anxiety only 50% as great as in all the studies
taken together. In other words, these techniques had seemed
to be more effective in the weaker studies than they actually
turned out to be when investigated in more rigorous studies.
With the Transcendental Meditation technique, however, the
results held steady. In the well-designed studies, in fact, the
reduction of anxiety by Transcendental Meditation was
slightly greater. When Dr. Eppley restricted his analysis to
only the best studies, this is to say, Transcendental Meditation
reduced anxiety more than four times as well as all other
techniques.

Because Transcendental Meditation was the first technique
to be scientifically tested, and has always received the most
publicity, its research has always received the most scrutiny.
For this reason, Eppley made a selection of only those studies
that (1) were well designed, and (2) had been done by
researchers who were either neutral or actively hostile toward
Transcendental Meditation. He wanted only those studies
that were both rigorous and clearly objective. The results
indicated conclusively that the stress-reducing effects of
Transcendental Meditation were not the result of experi-
menter bias. In this selection of studies by neutral researchers,
the Transcendental Meditation technique was found to reduce anxiety about 20% more effectively than it did in all the
studies taken together.[9]

THE MOST CHALLENGING STRESS DISORDER

The worst type of stress that psychologists ordinarily en-
counter in their patients is known as Post Traumatic Stress
Disorder. The best-known example of this is exhibited by a
high percentage of veterans of the Vietnam War. The hor-

rendous experiences undergone by some of these men created lasting trauma in their psychological make-up. These deep stresses still torment many veterans. They show up as severe anxiety, depression, emotional numbness, problems with alcohol and drugs, and/or inability to hold a job or maintain a family life. This post traumatic stress suffered by Vietnam veterans has proven extremely resistant to treatment. Some of these men have seen psychologists and attended counseling groups for many years, with little improvement.

Because of the severity of the problem, psychiatrist James Brooks, who worked at the Vietnam Veterans Outreach Center in Denver, Colorado, decided to test Transcendental Meditation as a treatment. Dr. Brooks reasoned that if Transcendental Meditation really is a significant tool for stress reduction, it might be able to help these most difficult cases.

Dr. Brooks randomly assigned one group of veterans to the standard type of psychological counseling available at the outreach center, and a second group to Transcendental Meditation. He did a prospective, longitudinal study, with pre- and post-testing over a three-month period. He had no dropouts. As expected, the psychological counseling had little effect; psychologists have been frustrated by this problem for years. Transcendental Meditation, however, did produce a wide range of statistically significant effects. The meditation group enjoyed significant reductions in anxiety, depression, emotional numbness, alcohol consumption, insomnia, and family problems. These men also displayed significant improvement in the ability to gain and maintain employment.[10]

MEDITATION AND FREE RADICALS

Taken together, these studies on Transcendental Meditation's effect on stress promise a uniquely effective answer to the problem of free radicals. Exhaustive meta-analyses and prospective, random-assignment comparisons are the most effective tools available to make such a judgment. In this instance, a "real" meditation technique—one that comes from the world's oldest tradition of knowledge and produces a fourth state of consciousness—reduces stress and anxiety much more effectively than any other technique tested to date. Many researchers feel that meditation is simply relaxation, but the data indicate that a fourth state of consciousness reduces anxiety two to four times better than physical relaxation techniques. It appears that relaxation is not the single active ingredient in Transcendental Meditation.

The most important question still remains. Scientific evidence of decreased stress is not complete without further studies defining benefits. Specifically, if Transcendental Meditation produces significant reductions in stress, that should also lead to (1) significant reductions in free radicals, and (2) significant improvements in every category of health.

In collaboration with investigators at MIU in Fairfield, Iowa, we at Ohio State have checked for lower free radical levels in meditators. We ran blood tests to determine levels of lipid peroxide in elderly people who have practiced the Transcendental Meditation technique for many years. Some of these meditators have utilized other Maharishi Ayur-Ved strategies as well. Tests for lipid peroxide are commonly used as an overall test of free radical activity in the body, as we have seen; if lipids are being damaged, the assumption is that other free radical damage is also occurring at a roughly similar pace.

In oxygen-based life, of course, it is not possible or necessary to reduce free radicals to zero. It is a question of balance—of reducing free radical activity just enough that the body's repair mechanisms can successfully keep up with the damage.

When we performed the lipid peroxide test on experienced meditators, we found a significant decrease in free radical levels. The meditators were compared to controls who did not meditate, and there was no significant difference in the amount of fat in the diets of the two groups. Yet the meditators in the age group 60–69 years exhibited a level of circulating lipid peroxide that was 14.5% lower. In the age group 70–79 years, the level of lipid peroxide was 16.5% lower. Reductions of this magnitude could favorably tip the free radical balance in the body.

STRESS, FREE RADICALS, AND AGING

Do the expected health benefits actually appear? This is the most practical and meaningful question—and it has been answered by a large number of studies on Transcendental Meditation and health. Targeted studies on particular health problems have indicated that Transcendental Meditation decreases many major health risk factors: blood pressure,[11] cholesterol,[12] smoking,[13] alcohol use,[14] and drug abuse.[15]

These wide-ranging health benefits led Dr. R. Keith Wallace to examine the effects of Transcendental Meditation on the aging process. As we have seen, aging can be defined most practically as (1) increased vulnerability to disease and (2) decreased capacity for physical function. Many free radical researchers have speculated that reduced free radical levels should slow both aspects of the aging process. Dr. Wallace decided to test physical functioning of the elderly.

Throughout most of this century, a standard test has been administered to hundreds of thousands of people that measures basic physiological functions—including near-point vision, auditory discrimination, and blood pressure. This test helped lead to the concept of *biological age* as distinct from *chronological age*. Biological age measures age in terms of physical function. Chronological age measures age in terms of years. A spry great-grandfather may have a biological age younger than his chronological age.

Dr. Wallace applied this standard test to people who practice Transcendental Meditation. His study statistically controlled for the effects of diet and exercise. As compared to normal values established over many years, those who had practiced Transcendental Meditation for up to five years had an average biological age five years younger than their chronological age. Those who had meditated over five years had an average biological age 12 years younger.[16] As Dr. Wallace noted, after years of meditation many of the subjects displayed a biological age that was younger than the chronological age they were on the day they learned to meditate. We have seen that reducing free radical damage can tip the body's internal balance and allow repair mechanisms to get ahead of ongoing damage. This should result in more youthful functioning. This study indicates that, with effective stress reduction, such a dramatic internal rebalancing may be possible.

A comparison on the elderly: Dr. Wallace's study was corroborated by a Harvard University study conducted by psychologists Charles Alexander and Ellen Langer on elderly residents of a nursing home. This study compared three types of meditation and relaxation techniques with a no-treatment control group. The residents, with an average age of 81 years, were randomly assigned to the four groups. The study lasted three years altogether, and showed that residents in the Transcendental Meditation group had the greatest reductions in stress and blood pressure. They were also the only group in which no one died during the study, although the average mortality rate in non-participating residents during those three years was more than one-third.[17]

Preserving hormones: A study published in the *Journal of Behavioral Medicine* and conducted by Dr. Jay Glaser, Medical Director of the Maharishi Ayur-Ved Health Center in Lancaster, Massachusetts, has also indicated that Transcendental Meditation may slow the aging process. Aging is partially caused by a reduction in hormone secretion. Without certain hormones, the body withers. We have discussed Richard Cutler's theory that reduced hormonal secretions may be due to cell dysdifferentiation caused by free radical damage. The same effect could be caused by atherosclerosis in the blood vessels leading to the hypothalamus, pituitary, and other glands. If stress creates free radicals, and free radicals reduce the level of hormones, then Transcendental Meditation should serve to maintain high levels of such hormones.

This has been tested with respect to one of the body's most significant and abundant hormones, dehydroepiandrosterone sulfate (DHEA-S). In a young adult, DHEA-S is the most abundant hormone in the body—but the levels decline rapidly with age. Men who maintain relatively high levels of DHEA-S have been shown to have less atherosclerosis and heart disease, and lower mortality rates from all causes. Women with high levels of DHEA-S are known to have less breast cancer and osteoporosis. Whereas the stress hormone cortisol leads to the breakdown of muscle tissue (to provide fuel for energy), DHEA-S leads to the build-up of muscle tissue. Influenced by DHEA-S, the body continues to build, instead of wasting away.

This study compared DHEA-S levels in the blood of 423 people who practiced Transcendental Meditation as compared to 1,253 healthy people who did not. The ages ranged from 20 to 81 years. Results were gathered in five-year age ranges. The effects of diet, obesity, and exercise were statistically ruled out. The results were consistent with Dr. Wallace's study. Depending on the age range, people who practiced Transcendental Meditation had levels of DHEA-S that were as high as members of the control group who were five to ten years younger.[18]

DECREASED HEALTH CARE COSTS

Do these effects really translate into improved health? After all, one of the best ways to demonstrate that aging has been slowed is to show that sickness has decreased. The overall effects of Transcendental Meditation on health have been shown most definitively by two studies of health insurance statistics. The first study was published in the journal *Psychosomatic Medicine* in 1987. Over a five-year period, this study tracked 2000 people all across the country who practiced Transcendental Meditation. The data was collected by an insurance company. The statistics from the meditation group were compared to a control group selected by the insurance company to match the Transcendental Meditation group for age, education, profession, and other variables.

The overall result was that, compared to the control group, the Transcendental Meditation group went to the hospital 56% less often.[19] In the Transcendental Meditation group, health insurance utilization was lower in all age groups, but the differences were largest in the older groups—where disease usually manifests most frequently. Moreover, the Transcendental Meditation group needed less medical assistance in every category of disease recorded by the insurance company. The statistics also indicated that the reduced usage of medical care was not due to a bias against doctors and hospitals. In fact, there was one category in which the meditating group used medical services slightly more than the controls: childbirth. Apparently, the meditators would go to the hospital if they needed to—but their need simply declined.

These statistics were gathered from the insurance company by meditation researcher Dr. David Orme-Johnson. Was there any flaw in the research design which could have accounted for such dramatic results? One possible criticism is that it was not a prospective study; it did not measure the subjects before they began Transcendental Meditation. In theory, at least, these people may have been extremely healthy before they began Transcendental Meditation.

A replication: To fill this gap, an MIU Ph.D. candidate, Robert Herron, undertook another study of insurance statistics. Herron took his data on Canadian citizens and obtained it from the Canadian government. Because Canada has national cradle-to-grave health care coverage, the government has data on every health care expenditure incurred by every citizen. It was possible to trace people's records back years before they learned Transcendental Meditation, then look for any changes that occurred as they learned and continued to meditate.

The study was also significant because it tracked not just health care utilization, but actual health care costs as well. Skyrocketing health care costs pose a severe threat to economic viability. Prior to this study, no research project had found a program that could reduce health care costs long-term. Some programs helped contain costs—helped to keep the upward spiral of prices from increasing so rapidly. But nothing had ever brought costs down on a sustainable basis.

That situation has now changed. All of the research on Transcendental Meditation has been summed up in dollars and cents. Herron found that, in the years before they learned Transcendental Meditation, the subjects' health care costs averaged the same as for all people in their age range. They were not a self-selected group of outstandingly healthy people. Once they began to meditate, however, their health care costs began to decline—an average of 10% each year.

The reductions were most dramatic among people who had previously shown the highest pattern of health care costs. The total group was divided into thirds, and in the third which had been to doctors and the hospital most frequently, the practice of Transcendental Meditation reduced health care costs by 18% a year—54% in three years. Among the elderly, the decline was slightly greater, 19% a year, 57% in three years. (These declines are inflation adjusted. Since health care costs were rising rapidly each year, the actual cost savings were considerably greater.)

COMBINED BENEFITS OF MAHARISHI AYUR-VED

Few people want to give up the high-tech advances that define modern life. But the health care crisis is sending us a wake-up call. We can no longer afford to pay for the amount of sickness we inflict on ourselves with our stressful lifestyles. We appear to be at a crossroads. Either we renounce progress, and return to a simpler, less stressful lifestyle, or we develop the ability to withstand stress without mass producing free radicals. Either we find a way to reduce the damage caused by stress, or we watch as it breaks down our health—and our national economy.

Herron's study clearly indicated that stress can be reduced—meaning that free radicals can be controlled. For the first time, a systematic program had been identified that could reduce actual dollars spent on health care. Moreover, the reductions clearly began when the people started to practice Transcendental Meditation. For the first time, beleaguered governments and corporations, under free radical attack and staggering beneath the crushing weight of health care costs, had a scientifically verified option to fend off free radicals and slash their health care outlays year after year.[20]

It appears that we can turn the tide of battle against stress and free radicals. We can use a simple meditation technique to dissolve stress and negate its free radical-creating effect.

Combined with the results on Maharishi Amrit Kalash, moreover, these findings suggest that we can live our lives with a completely different internal chemistry. It appears possible to decisively alter the free radical balance in the body. The Transcendental Meditation technique slows the creation of free radicals. Maharishi Amrit Kalash scavenges those that do get created with unique efficiency. The scientific evidence on both approaches shows that, as the pressure of constant free radical damage eases, physical health improves in many different ways.

The combined effects have been tested in one of the most significant research studies I have encountered. It is a third study of insurance statistics, completed just as this book was going to press. Dr. David Orme-Johnson collected insurance data for a seven-year period on all the faculty and staff of Maharishi International University in Fairfield, Iowa. This study included a significant new element. The people at Maharishi International University not only practiced Transcendental Meditation. Most of them also used advanced meditation techniques known as the TM-Sidhi program, and many used Maharishi Amrit Kalash regularly. Some also took advantage of additional prevention-oriented programs offered by Maharishi Ayur-Ved (see Chapter Nine for details on the many approaches of Maharishi Ayur-Ved). This study, therefore, was a comparative test of the disease-prevention power of Maharishi Ayur-Ved as a whole.

Like the study comparing Maharishi Amrit Kalash with other anti-oxidants, this study produced the type of results rare in medical science. This was not just another laboratory study, finding results in a test tube that might or might not recur in living human beings. Nor was it an isolated study of one symptom or disease that might or might not generalize to other problems. This was a study that went straight to the bottom line: When a group of people control free radicals with Maharishi Ayur-Ved, what happens to overall health?

The earlier studies had shown that Transcendental Meditation by itself could reduce hospital utilization by about half. The new study showed that adding MAK and other aspects of Maharishi Ayur-Ved helped cut that rate by more than half again. Over the seven years, comparing the MIU group to all the other Iowans insured by the same company, the MIU group was hospitalized for illness and surgery 86% less.[21]

This means the MIU group was six times less likely to fall seriously ill. Once again, hospitalization for childbirth was about equal between the two groups, indicating that the re-duced hospitalization for the MIU group was not due to a bias against hospitals. Moreover, all subjects were Iowans, mean-ing that risk factors for disease were roughly equal. A study comparing Iowans against people from New York or Los Angeles would be less compelling; people in large cities are arguably exposed to more environmental health risks.

To tighten the match with the control group even more, Dr. Orme-Johnson also compared MIU's faculty and staff with data from the same insurance company on the faculty and staff of 18 other small colleges, from small towns, in Iowa. More than 5,000 people were involved, and these two groups were a nearly exact match for age, sex, race, education, pro-fession, environment, and every other significant variable. The data was independently collected by the insurance company itself. The result was virtually identical: The MIU group was hospitalized for illness and surgery 82% less.[22]

A NEW MEDICAL ERA

In terms of my own biography and Indian heritage, these findings have been both startling and, I must admit, quietly gratifying. When young, I deliberately left the ayurvedic tradition of my homeland. I forged a career in the West, in Western medicine and medical research. Now the scientific skills I mastered in that career have allowed me to make a contribution toward the rediscovery of ayurveda—and its unique effectiveness for prevention of disease.

In my life, I have experienced a sudden and dramatic transformation. Even five or six years ago I would never have imagined the breakthroughs that were coming. The research on Maharishi Amrit Kalash began in 1987, the same year that the major comparative and insurance studies on Transcendental Meditation began to appear in academic journals. In scarcely more than half a decade, my entire medical outlook has been revised.

I am convinced the transformation is just as great for the whole of the medical world. A new era is opening in medical history. Free radicals are implicated in much of aging and degenerative disease. Maharishi Amrit Kalash and Transcendental Meditation control free radicals and produce spectacular long-range improvements in health. The dual discovery has led to a statistically measurable transformation of the possibilities of human life.

As we saw in Part One, mainstream medical investigators are speculating that the average life span can be increased to 120–150 years. A few optimists have mentioned 200 years. But no one really knows what is possible if free radical damage is sufficiently controlled. Certainly the implications of recent studies for both health and longevity are significantly more optimistic than any researcher could have dreamed ten years ago. Even in our highly stressful society, it appears that good health and youthful functioning can be retained far longer than we had previously hoped.

The ayurvedic tradition itself makes the boldest claim: *Ayurved amritanam* ("Ayurved is for immortality"). Modern experience may not have prepared us for such a statement, but neither had modern experience prepared us for the research findings on free radicals and free radical management.

It seems that those of us alive today have the chance to find out what no generation in recorded history has yet known— what life is like with free radical damage under much better control.

FROM FACTS TO THEORY

There is yet one further step to take in this book. Until now we have focused almost exclusively on research facts and figures. But a new paradigm demands more than objective evidence. It also requires a new theoretical understanding. When the Wright brothers were pushing their first biplane down the slope at Kitty Hawk, many people felt that heavier-than-air machines could never fly. They did not understand the concepts of air flow and dynamic lift that explain why airplanes larger and heavier than most single family dwellings plow into the sky routinely.

Such a theoretical breakthrough is also required to explain why Maharishi Ayur-Ved works so well. The approaches of Maharishi Ayur-Ved, including Maharishi Amrit Kalash and Transcendental Meditation, stem from a tradition that pre-dates the age of science by thousands of years. Why is it then, that once the latest science had come up with a unified mechanism for disease and aging, it turned out that ancient methods counteract that mechanism most effectively? To put the question more colloquially, what did the ayurvedic vaidyas know thousands of years ago that we don't know today?

These are questions we will address in Part Three. They will take this book in a totally new direction—but the direction is important. For reasonable people to accept that airplanes can fly, experiment should be backed by theory. For reasonable people to accept that ancient technologies most effectively meet the free radical challenge, the information presented in the first two parts of this book should be backed by theoretical justification.

FROM BODY TO MIND

To lead up to this theory-building most logically, we should look briefly at an aspect of the research on Transcendental Meditation which we have glossed over until now. Our focus has been on free radicals, and thus on the stress reduction afforded by the Transcendental Meditation technique. We have covered research showing that Transcendental Meditation produces a unique style of rest and relaxation in the body. But we have paid little attention to what happens in the brain and mind. This is typical of most medical analyses of meditation; until recently, the focus has been almost solely on physical relaxation.

Maharishi, however, describes Transcendental Meditation's effects in terms of a fourth state of consciousness. He maintains that regular meditation leads to the "evolution of consciousness"—the unfoldment of full mental potential. We have also seen that Maharishi Amrit Kalash affects the molecular operation of the brain and limbic system—altering consciousness as well as physiology. From this perspective, research on Transcendental Meditation's effect on the brain and mental functioning could well be significant—even for physical health.

Scientific studies in this area have investigated three factors:

1. Brain functioning during meditation.

2. Brain functioning after meditation.

3. Mental and psychological benefits of meditation.

During meditation: We have already seen that, during the practice of Transcendental Meditation, blood flow to the brain increases markedly. Other research shows that unique changes also appear in brain wave patterns. For example, there is a marked increase in alpha power in the frontal regions of the brain—a much greater increase than occurs in ordinary eyes-closed resting.[23] Years of research have shown that such alpha waves ordinarily indicate a relaxed but alert style of mental functioning.

In addition, many studies have reported that the brain appears to "get itself together." During Transcendental Meditation, there is an increase in brain wave *coherence*. In the frontal regions of the brain, the electrical activity becomes more orderly and synchronous.[24] The brain begins to function in an integrated style in the frontal and central regions—a pattern of brain wave coherence never previously seen. All these changes together amount to a unique pattern of brain activity not found in any of the three common states of consciousness (waking, sleeping, dreaming). They are thus consistent with Maharishi's description of a fourth state of consciousness.

After meditation: Research has also shown that after meditation the patterns of coherent brain wave activity tend to persist.[25] There are also indications that brain processing speed has improved. Two recent studies have measured changes in *evoked potentials* (electrical activity in the brain evoked by a stimulus such as a mild shock). These studies show that when experienced meditators work on a challenging mental problem, their brains react significantly more quickly than is seen in non-meditating controls.[26] Another study has shown that experienced meditators choose and react more quickly in a complex reaction time test which measures the speed with which electrical signals are processed in the brain.[27] Finally, biochemical measurements have indicated that people who practice Transcendental Meditation have higher baseline levels of serotonin, the neurotransmitter that correlates positively with upbeat emotions that range from comfort to exhilaration.[28]

Long-range benefits: If you tune up an automobile engine, it delivers more horsepower. If you tune up the brain with meditation, it apparently delivers improved mental functioning. The mental benefits of Transcendental Meditation have been depicted in a long series of studies. People who practice the Transcendental Meditation technique display increased intelligence,[29] enhanced creativity,[30] improved memory,[31] and improved college grades.[32] In addition, there is a marked improvement in psychological health and maturity, including increased self-confidence and self-esteem, enhancement of the ability to relate to other people, and improvements in overall psychological development.[33]

It is common sense that brain activity relates to consciousness. It is plausible that the "evolution of consciousness" can be measured in terms of mental abilities and psychological maturity. Given these assumptions, a large number of research studies indicate that Maharishi's theories of consciousness have a scientific foundation. There does appear to be a fourth state of consciousness—measurable through changes in the functioning of the brain and body. There does appear to be evolution of consciousness—measurable in terms of increased intelligence, creativity, and psychological maturity.

According to these findings, Maharishi's Transcendental Meditation technique tunes the brain to a new, and apparently better, style of functioning. The result is improved mental performance. A more efficient central processing chip improves computer output. A brain cultured to more integrated functioning improves mental output. No similar pattern of brain refinement and mental improvement has been shown for any other meditation or relaxation technique.

For our considerations in Part Three, these findings are highly significant. They indicate that improvements in physical health produced by Transcendental Meditation are tied to parallel improvements in the quality of consciousness. We want to determine how ancient techniques fight free radicals so much more effectively than modern approaches. In Maharishi's view, as we will see, the answer comes down to one word: consciousness.

Notes

1. Levine SA, Kidd PM, *Antioxidant Adaptation: Its Role in Free Radical Pathology* (Biocurrents Division, Allergy Research Group, San Leandro, 1986), p. 241-2

2. Oates RM Jr., *Celebrating the Dawn* (G.P. Putnam's Sons, New York, 1976), p. 29

3. Murphy M, Donovan S, *The Physical and Psychological Effects of Meditation: A Review of Contemporary Meditation Research with a Comprehensive Bibliography 1931-1988* (Esalen, San Rafael, 1988)

4. Jevning R, et al, *Phys and Behav* 29(1982): 343-8

5. Jevning R, *The Physiologist* 21(1978): 60

6. Dillbeck MC, et al, *Amer Psychol* 42(1987): 879-81

7. Ibid

8. Eppley K, et al, *J Clin Psychol* 45(1989): 957-74

9. Ibid

10. Brooks JS, Scarano T, *J Counsel Devt* 65(1985): 212-5

11. Wallace RK, et al, *Psychosom Med* 45(1983): 41-6

12. Cooper MJ, Aygen MM, *J Human Stress* 5(1979): 24-7

13. Monahan RJ, *Int'l J Addictions* 12(1977): 729-54

14. Shafii M, et al, *Amer J Psychia* 132(1975): 942-5

15. Gelderloos P, et al, *Int'l J Addictions* 26(1991): 293-325

16. Wallace RK, et al, *Int'l J Neurosci* 16(1982): 53-8

17. Alexander CN, et al, *J Personality Soc Psych* 57(1989): 950-64

18. Glaser JL, et al, *J Behav Med* 15(4)(1992): 327-41

19. Orme-Johnson D, *Psychosom Med* 49(1987): 493-507

20. Herron RE, *The Impact of Transcendental Meditation Practice on Medical Expenditures*, A Dissertation Submitted to the Graduate School of Maharishi Int'l University (August, 1992)

21. Orme-Johnson DW, presented at the Annual Conference of the American Journal of Health Promotion, Atlanta, February 22-26, 1993

22. Orme-Johnson DW, *Journal of the Iowa Academy of Science* 95(1988): A56 (Abstract)

23. Wallace RK, et al, *Am J Phys* 221(1971): 795-9

24. Badawi K, et al, *Psychosom Med* 46(1984): 267-76

25. Dillbeck MC, Bronson EC, *Int'l J Neurosci* 14(1981): 147-51

26. Goddard PH, *Psychophysiol* 26(1989): S29 (Abstract)

27. Cranson R, et al, *Personality and Indiv Diff* 12(1991): 1105-16

28. Bujatti M, Reiderer P, *J Neural Transm* 39(1976): 257-67; Walton KG, et al, *Trans Am Soc Neurochem* 14(1983): 199

29. Cranson, *Personality* (see note 26); Aron A, *Coll Stu J* 15(1981): 140-6

30. Travis F, *J Creat Behav* 13(1979): 169-80

31. Dillbeck MC, et al, *Mem and Cog* 10(1982): 207-15

32. Kember P, *British J Ed Psych* 55(1985): 164-6

33. Alexander CN, et al, *J Soc Behav Personality* 6(1991): 189-247; Alexander CN, Langer EJ, eds., *Higher Stages of Human Development: Perspectives on Adult Growth* (Oxford University Press, New York, 1990), pp. 286-341; Seeman W, et al, *J Couns Psych* 19(1972): 184-7

PART THREE

The Consciousness
Paradigm

CHAPTER SEVEN

Living in Tune with Nature's Intelligence

The damage caused by free radicals can be markedly reduced. Based on the research evidence available right now, human beings should be able to live longer and much healthier lives.

But the need for a new theory of health seems obvious. Why should traditional approaches fight free radicals more effectively than modern ones? It may not seem to make sense. Most of us are used to thinking of traditional medicine as folk medicine, unsystematic and unscientific, altogether too close to the quaint nostrums our grandmothers used to recommend. We live, after all, in an age of science. We are used to seeking knowledge through objective investigation—through laboratory experimentation. Obviously, ayurvedic medicine did not begin that way.

In this section of the book, we will deal with this issue. As the Introduction pointed out, the health breakthroughs we have seen in the last few chapters depend on a dual discovery. The first part of this discovery is the free radical paradigm: Cellular damage done by ravenous oxygen-based molecules causes much of disease and aging. The second part is a consciousness-based system of natural health care: Free radicals can be controlled most effectively by health care that connects body with mind.

The research evidence on Maharishi Ayur-Ved has given indications of these mind-body effects. Maharishi Amrit Kalash, for instance, is a physical substance. However, by supplying biochemicals that react with brain receptors that correlate with a more relaxed and positive mood, it affects consciousness. The Transcendental Meditation technique works in the opposite direction. It is a purely mental technique. However, by creating a relaxed and positive state of mind, it breaks the stress syndrome and generates a different pattern of biochemicals in the body. MAK, in other words, works from body to mind, Transcendental Meditation from mind to body. According to the research evidence, this integrated approach works much more effectively than mechanical antioxidants that can only operate molecule-on-molecule.

It is a body of scientific evidence that requires a new theoretical explanation. Mind and body certainly seem connected—primarily through the limbic system—but a profound conceptual understanding is lacking. How can consciousness, with no material existence, interact with the solid substance of the physical body? How can the non-material affect the material? To provide an answer, we need a consciousness-based paradigm for physical health.

These are issues that will be explored in this chapter and the next. They can first be addressed by a practical question: How did vaidyas, thousands of years before the age of science, discover health care technologies that science has now proven so effective? It's a puzzle worth our attention—because the method of gaining knowledge tells a great deal about the knowledge discovered. The factual information known to modern science is based on the reductionist approach of objective investigation. But the original ayurvedic vaidyas did not use objective investigation. Instead, they used systematic techniques for *subjective* investigation. They didn't look outside, at the world around them. They turned within, to the most profound levels of their own consciousness. They obtained their information by cognizing it directly, complete and in detail, deep within their own minds.

THE SUBJECTIVE APPROACH TO KNOWLEDGE

This is the conception that has been passed down from generation to generation, for thousands of years. It is said that the whole of ayurvedic knowledge was seen at once, by a sage named Bharadwaja, through the use of a systematic technology for subjective investigation. These traditional stories about Bharadwaja may sound unscientific on first hearing but the ancient stories give details about the approach used. They paint a picture that is clear enough to investigate within the Western scientific tradition.

In the ancient tales, Bharadwaja and many of his colleagues were depicted as deeply committed to improving human health and easing both physical and mental suffering. They saw illness increasing in their society and wanted to do something about it. Their resolve became so strong that they determined to uncover the deepest truths of human physiology and perfect health.

To seek useful knowledge, Bharadwaja was joined by scores of the most accomplished meditation experts of his time. These were great sages, enlightened masters with highly refined awareness. Full of the desire to ease human suffering, these sages sat with Bharadwaja to practice group dynamics of consciousness—long sessions of group meditation. As told in the stories that have come down to us, in the intensely coherent atmosphere created by these powerful minds all meditating together, Bharadwaja was able to directly cognize the essence of ayurveda. The insights that came to him were written down as *Charak Samhita*, still the essential textbook of ayurvedic medicine.

In this story there seems to be no trace of the scientific approach. Bharadwaja used no test tubes, no machinery, no double-blind trials—no objective investigation at all. The whole process was completely subjective, deep within consciousness. In the Western scientific tradition, there at first appears to be no explanation for this phenomenon. The Vedic tradition, however, does offer a systematic explanation. It is not a theory widely understood in this scientific age—and yet it correlates with the most profound thoughts and experiences of many leading scientists. This explanation provides the basis for the explorations of this chapter. It also provides a consciousness paradigm for physical health.

THE CONSCIOUSNESS PARADIGM

The Vedic tradition understands that nature is not fundamentally objective. It is not based on material objects. Rather, the most fundamental reality is said to be completely subjective—an unbounded and eternal field of pure, abstract intelligence, or consciousness. When Maharishi Mahesh Yogi speaks on this topic, he indicates that the field of pure intelligence permeates everything—like a vast ocean of consciousness. What we see as the material world is, in reality, waves, or fluctuations, or impulses, of this underlying non-material field of pure consciousness. What we ourselves are, mind and body, is intelligence in motion.

In this Vedic understanding, if the human mind becomes still and pure enough, it can contact this pure field of consciousness at the basis of the physical world. It can settle down to become directly aware of the finest fluctuations of its own intelligence—said to be the same as the finest fluctuations of the intelligence in nature. Human intelligence and nature's intelligence are one and the same. The human mind can directly cognize even the subtlest laws of nature.

To people raised and trained in the tradition of objective, scientific investigation, this may all sound quite unlikely. But there are at least two reasons to pay these understandings closer attention. First, of course, the scientific evidence reviewed in this book has upheld the effectiveness of the ayurvedic techniques first discovered through such subjective investigation. Second, as we will see in this chapter, the understandings and techniques of Vedic sages and modern scientists are not really that far apart. The Vedic understanding of nature, for example, parallels the discoveries of modern physics. As this chapter shows, modern physics has caused many leading scientists to decide that the physical world actually *is* based on intelligence or consciousness. And despite the apparent commitment of Western science to logical, objective investigation, many of the most important discoveries in modern science have been made just as Bharadwaja made his —as sudden, all-at-once intuitions or cognitions. A direct, subjective route to truth is not confined to ayurvedic vaidyas.

We will start our explorations by examining this phenomenon of direct intuition or cognition. As we progress, we will confront some of the most profound theories of modern science. These ideas have been thoroughly discussed by leading physicists and mathematicians of our century and I will rely throughout this discussion on quotations from experts in these fields. We will find that the latest breakthroughs in mathematics and physics can help make sense of subjective investigation. They can also make a major difference in human health.

Pasteur discovered the health of the entire human body could be explained at the level of single cells. Recent free radical research has shown that disruptions at the level of the cell can be explained by going deeper, to the level of the molecule. Now we will see that the molecular level of human health can be explained by going to the deepest level of nature, the level of unbounded, non-material, quantum mechanical fields.

INTUITION IN OBJECTIVE SCIENCE

To begin this quest, we can start with the phenomenon of sudden, direct inspiration, or intuition, or cognition. Scientific discoveries are often thought to result from a laborious gathering of facts, from precise experimentation and strict logic. Scientific knowledge is supposedly built up brick by brick through objective means. In fact, however, many of the most significant breakthroughs in the history of science have suddenly blossomed in someone's mind unbidden, all at once. As we all have experienced at some point in our lives, "The idea just came to me." The French mathematician Henri Poincaré, for example, is well known for his experiences of spontaneous inner problem-solving. He has described one of his most important discoveries as follows:

> . . . I left Caen, where I was living, to go on a geologic excursion under the auspices of the School of Mines. The incidents of the travel made me forget my mathematical work. Having reached Coutances, we entered an omnibus to go to some place or other. At the moment when I put my foot on the step, the idea came to me, without anything in my former thoughts seeming to have paved the way for it, that the transformations I had used to define the Fuchsian functions were identical with those of non-Euclidean geometry. I did not verify the idea; I should not have had time, as upon taking my seat in the omnibus, I went on with a conversation already commenced, but I felt a perfect certainty. On my return to Caen, for convenience sake, I verified the result at my leisure.[1]

A second example comes from a leading astrophysicist of our own time, Fred Hoyle:

> As the miles slipped by I turned the quantum mechanical problem . . . over in my mind, in the hazy way I normally have in thinking mathematics in my head. Normally, I have to write things down on paper, and then fiddle with the equations and integrals as best I can. But somewhere on Bowes Moor my awareness of the mathematics clarified, not a little, not even a lot, but as if a huge brilliant light had suddenly been switched on. How long did it take to become totally convinced that the problem was solved? Less than five sec-

onds. It only remained to make sure that before the clarity faded I had enough of the essential steps stored safely in my recallable memory. It is indicative of the measure of certainty I felt that in the ensuing days I didn't trouble to commit anything to paper. When ten days or so later I returned to Cambridge I found it possible to write out the thing without difficulty.[2]

Finally, in the same vein, from one of the most influential mathematical physicists, Roger Penrose of Oxford University:

A colleague had been visiting from the USA and he was engaging me in voluble conversation on a quite different topic as we walked down the street approaching my office in Birkbeck College in London. The conversation stopped momentarily as we crossed a side road, and resumed again at the other side. Evidently, during those few moments, an idea occurred to me, but then the ensuing conversation blotted it from my mind! Later in the day, after my colleague had left, I returned to my office. I remember having an odd feeling of elation that I could not account for. I began going through in my mind all the various things that had happened to me during the day, in an attempt to find what it was that had caused this elation. After eliminating numerous inadequate possibilities, I finally brought to mind the thought that I had while crossing the street—a thought which had momentarily elated me by providing the solution to the problem that had been milling around at the back of my head! Apparently, it was the needed criterion—that I subsequently called a 'trapped surface'—and then it did not take me long to form the outline of a proof of the theorem that I had been looking for.[3]

Stories like these abound in the history of science and mathematics. In 1865, for example, Friedrich August Kekule von Stradonitz suddenly saw the answer to a problem that had been vexing him for seven years. He had a vision of the benzene ring (six carbon atoms joined together in a hexagon) while riding half asleep in a horse-drawn coach. In 1764, the Scottish engineer James Watt invented a radically improved steam engine in an instant while out for a Sunday afternoon walk. In 1843, Irish mathematician William Rowan Hamilton realized the solution to a knotty problem (he had to grasp that there were conditions under which "p x q" does not equal "q x p") while walking his wife to town. In 1921, German physiologist Otto Loewi awoke one night at 3 a.m. with a clear idea for an experiment that would solve the neurochemical problem he was facing. He wrote it down, but in the morning, he couldn't read his writing or remember the idea. When the idea woke him again the next night, he dressed, went to his lab, performed the experiment before dawn, and obtained results that eventually won him the Nobel prize.[4]

ANALYSIS OF INTUITION

These experiences of scientific inspiration or intuition, coming suddenly and spontaneously while the conscious mind is at ease (or even asleep), are so common that they have been codified into a system. The mathematician J.E. Littlewood identifies four states: (1) preparation, when the mind deliberately ponders the problem, (2) incubation, when the conscious thinking mind goes on to other things, (3) illumination, usually in a period of relaxation when the mind appears to be occupied with other topics, and (4) verification, which can be done by anyone competent in the field.[5]

The common thread for the inspiration itself is that it comes instantly, all at once, with no warning. Says the 19th century mathematical genius Carl Gauss of such an intuitive leap: "Like a sudden flash of lightning, the riddle happened to be solved. I myself cannot say what was the conducting thread which connected what I previously knew with what made my success possible."[6]

Science writer Isaac Asimov pondered the apparently embarrassing implications of this sudden Aha! experience. Science is supposed to be logical and systematic. But major discoveries are often sudden intuitions. As he says,

> How often does this 'eureka phenomenon' happen? How often is there this flash of deep insight during a moment of relaxation, this triumphant cry of 'I've got it! I've got it!' which must surely be a

moment of the purest ecstasy this sorry world can afford? I wish there were some way we could tell. I suspect that in the history of science it happens often. . . . But the world is in a conspiracy to hide the fact. Scientists are wedded to reason, to the meticulous working out of consequences from assumptions, to the careful organization of experiments designed to check those consequences. If a certain line of experiments ends nowhere, it is omitted from the final report. If an inspired guess turns out to be correct, it is not reported as an inspired guess. . . . The scientist actually becomes ashamed of having what we might call a revelation, as though to have one is to betray reason . . . .[7]

The history of science leaves no doubt that important ideas can come to the mind spontaneously. Even in the tradition of objective investigation, there is clear evidence for a subjective route to truth. But what accounts for these sudden inspirations? Where does the mind get these ideas? Some observers, including Asimov, speculate that there is not much mystery. A sudden solution, these people say, comes from nothing other than rational, logical thought—but rational, logical thought that is conducted subconsciously and automatically. Many others, however, feel that such an explanation doesn't square with the experience. The inspired ideas come all at once and whole, often as a visual image, with a sense of certainty that is utterly devoid of proof or intervening logical steps. The logical proof, in fact, must be carried out afterward.

THE PLATONIC EXPLANATION

To explain this facility of the mind, Roger Penrose, the Oxford mathematical physicist, has recently re-enlivened an idea first put forward by Plato 2,500 years ago. In his recent influential book, *The Emperor's New Mind*, Penrose restates Plato's argument that mathematical concepts and structures (what Plato called *forms*) exist in their ideal state in a non-material realm that is open to experience by the human intellect. It is possible, for example, to imagine a perfect square, two inches on each side. In Plato's view, the mind can "see" this square, more perfect than any that can be drawn in the real world, because the form of the square exists within the nature of intelligence. It is independent of any particular mind, and available to all. The same thing is true, Plato and Penrose say, of even the most complex mathematical structures. Penrose explains:

> I imagine that whenever the mind perceives a mathematical idea, it makes contact with Plato's world of mathematical concepts. . . . When one 'sees' a mathematical truth, one's consciousness breaks through into this world of ideas, and makes direct contact with it.... When mathematicians communicate, this is made possible by each one having a direct route to truth, the consciousness of each being in a position to perceive mathematical truths directly, through this process of 'seeing'. (Indeed, often this act of perception is accompanied by words like 'Oh, I see'!) Since each can make contact with Plato's world directly, they can more readily communicate with each other than one might have expected. The mental images that each one has, when making this Platonic contact, might be rather different in each case, but communication is possible because each is directly in contact with the same eternally existing Platonic world! According to this view, the mind is always capable of this direct contact. But only a little may come through at a time. Mathematical discovery consists of broadening the area of contact. . . . All the information was there all the time. It was just a matter of putting things together and 'seeing' the answer! This is very much in accordance with Plato's own idea that (say mathematical) discovery is just a form of remembering![8]

Other researchers make similar points. Mathematician Rudy Rucker posits a "Mindscape," a world of the intelligence common to all. As Rucker says, "A person who does mathematical research is an explorer of the Mindscape in much the same way that Armstrong, Livingstone, or Cousteau are explorers of the physical features of our Universe. . . . Just as we all share the same Universe, we all share the same Mindscape."[9]

The existence of this Mindscape can help explain sudden intuitions or cognitions. If mathematical forms pre-exist in

Plato's realm of pure intelligence, then the mind can suddenly stumble upon one. It can "see" it whole. Paul Erdös, an eccentric and brilliant mathematician, is a traveling problem-solver who shows up suddenly at the doors of leading mathematicians worldwide, offering his temporary services to solve whatever problems are outstanding. He is famous for his ability to quickly intuit answers. He has published more than 1,000 papers, and frequently offers rewards to people who can write out the proofs to some of his more profound insights. When asked where he gets his ideas, he says "straight from the book." He elaborates that God has "a transfinite book of theorems in which the best proofs are written. And if he is well intentioned, he gives us the book for a moment."[10]

As physicist Paul Davies says of the astonishing theorems written by an untutored mathematical prodigy, Srinivasa Ramanujan, "It is very tempting to suppose that Ramanujan had a particular faculty that enabled him to view the mathematical Mindscape directly and vividly, and pluck out ready-made results at will."[11]

THE SUBJECTIVE IS OBJECTIVE

This Platonic notion of a realm of perfect mathematical structures accounts for the certainty which some people feel when they have sudden, intuitive flashes that produce new answers. Such intuitions may be subjective in the sense that they occur within the mind rather than in the world of material objects. But they may be considered objective in the sense that they are unchanging realities in the intellectual sphere. In Penrose's phrase, they are "mathematician-independent." Says Kurt Gödel, whose *incompleteness theorem* revolutionized mathematical theory in 1931:

> It by no means follows, however, that [intuitions], because they cannot be associated with actions of certain things upon our sense organs, are something purely subjective. . . . Rather, they too may represent an aspect of objective reality, but, as opposed to the sen-

sations, their presence in us may be due to another kind of relationship between ourselves and reality.[12]

INTELLIGENCE AND NATURAL LAW

Introducing the notion of "reality," as Gödel does, reminds us that there is another step to take in this logic. Mathematicians report having access to a Platonic realm of mathematical truths. But Bharadwaja's cognitions did not involve abstract math. They involved the real world—especially the physical body. Can intuition, direct subjective investigation within the Mindscape, produce valid knowledge about the outer, physical world?

One answer is that the laws which describe the outer, physical world are, in fact, purely mathematical in form. For example, Newton showed that the amount of force needed to accelerate a given mass can be calculated by the formula $F=ma$. Einstein showed that the amount of energy corresponding to mass is given by $E=mc^2$. All the laws of nature discovered by modern science can be written out in such mathematical formulas. As Galileo said at the dawn of the scientific era: "The book of nature is written in mathematical language."[13] Sir James Jeans, one of England's leading physicists of the twentieth century, commented that "the universe appears to have been designed by a pure mathematician."[14] In the words of physicist Paul Davies, who has become the premier translator of modern quantum mechanical discoveries into plain English, "Perhaps the greatest scientific discovery of all time is that nature is written in mathematical code. . . . Once we have cracked the code for some particular system, we can read nature like a book."[15]

The fit between pure mathematics and the laws of nature is so precise, in fact, that mathematicians often make discoveries that are only later found to describe some feature of the physical world. In a famous example, mathematicians Carl

Gauss and Bernhard Riemann worked out mathematics of curved surfaces in the 19th century which were later found to apply exactly in Einstein's geometrical theory of gravity. But why should this be? Why should abstract mathematical formulas, freely created within the human mind, match up so exactly with phenomena in the physical world? Why should the mathematicians' "independent world created out of pure intelligence," to take a phrase from British physicist Sir James Jeans,[16] precisely parallel the world constructed out of solid matter? It's such a puzzle that Nobel laureate Eugene Wigner speaks of "the unreasonable effectiveness of mathematics in the natural sciences,"[17] and Einstein commented that, "The only incomprehensible thing about the universe is that it is comprehensible."[18]

The most straightforward explanation for the math-physics match is that the intelligence within the human mind parallels exactly the intelligence displayed in the laws of nature. In the view of many physicists, such profound congruence could not be coincidence. As Penrose says,

> There must, instead, be some deep underlying reason for the accord between mathematics and physics, i.e. between Plato's world and the physical world. . . . The very precision of [the best scientific] theories has provided an almost abstract mathematical existence for actual physical reality. . . . This is perhaps the other side of the coin to the question of how abstract mathematical concepts can achieve an almost concrete reality in Plato's world. Perhaps, in some sense, the two worlds are actually the same?[19]

Heinrich Hertz, the physicist who first showed how to produce and investigate electric waves, commented on the ability of the human mind to create mathematical symbol systems that can predict the course of natural events: "A certain concordance must prevail between nature and our mind, or else this demand could not be satisfied."[20]

MATTER AND MIND

To many of the leading physicists of our time, however, the relationship between human intelligence and the natural world—between mind and matter—is much more intimate than mere correspondence. In this view, the parallels between mathematics and natural law result from a fundamental unity between the intelligence displayed in the human mind and the intelligence displayed in the natural world. Human intelligence corresponds with nature's intelligence because the two are, in fact, different aspects of one underlying reality.

This view contradicts the apparent distinction between mind and matter. It seems that nothing could unite such disparate phenomena. The mind is subjective. Matter is objective. The mind is the subject. Matter is the object. We have been talking of intelligence, of mind, but through most of the history of science, matter has been the dominant subject. A central premise of "objective" science, after all, is that objects exist. The essence of materialism is matter-realism. And solid matter would seem to provide a distinct barrier to the unity of human intelligence with nature's intelligence. There is one factor that needs to be taken into account, however. In the twentieth century, physicists have discovered that solid matter does not exist.

This is a discovery that has not yet made its way into popular thought. Certainly medical doctors treat the human body as though it were solid stuff—an extremely complex machine, perhaps, but understandable in terms of mere arrangements of matter. This understanding of the body, and the world around us, is still based on nineteenth-century physics—on Newtonian, or classical, physics—in which matter was considered fundamental. In the words of Werner Heisenberg, one of the twentieth-century pioneers who developed modern quantum mechanical physics:

The nineteenth century developed an extremely rigid frame for natural science which formed not only science but also the general outlook of great masses of people. . . . Matter was the primary reality. The progress of science was pictured as a crusade of conquest into the material world. . . . Mechanics was the methodological example for all science.[21]

It was, in fact, the very success of classical physics in the nineteenth century which biased the viewpoint of many who produced its greatest achievements. The success of objective investigation led some of these people to deny even the existence of subjective reality. As Nobel laureate Eugene Wigner said,

> Until not many years ago, the 'existence' of a mind or soul would have been passionately denied by most physical scientists. The brilliant successes of mechanistic and, more generally, macroscopic physics and of chemistry overshadowed the obvious fact that thoughts, desires, and emotions are not made of matter, and it was nearly universally accepted among physical scientists that there is nothing besides matter.[22]

In the twentieth century, deeper exploration into nature has revealed a deeper reality. Matter is made of atoms, atoms are made of sub-atomic "particles," and, as we have seen in Chapter Two, these sub-atomic building blocks of nature are not made of solid matter. There are no ultimate billiard balls, or building blocks. Instead, electrons, quarks, and other sub-atomic realities are nothing but non-material waves moving through non-material fields.

If you are afloat in the Pacific, the waves that pass may appear to have a separate and localized existence, but they are actually just fluctuations of the limitless ocean. In the same way, sub-atomic particles may sometimes appear to have a physical reality, but they are actually compact fluctuations in an unbounded, non-material field that extends throughout the universe. Physicist Fritjof Capra says, "Particles are merely local condensations of the field; concentrations of energy which come and go, thereby losing their individual character and dissolving into the underlying field."[23] Paul Davies reports that, "What we used to regard as solid objects are found to be a ghostly mosaic of quivering energy."[24] And Einstein summed up the discovery in unambiguous terms: "We may therefore regard matter as being constituted by the regions of space in which the field is extremely intense. . . . [T]here is no place in this new kind of physics both for the field and matter, for the field is the only reality."[25]

WHY THE WORLD SEEMS SOLID

"Solid matter" appears solid only at the macroscopic level of life—the level where we live. The illusion is created by our senses and by the electromagnetic force.

Our eyes are set to perceive nature only at a scale much larger than the sub-atomic reality. The retina of the eye registers electromagnetic waves reflecting from the environment, and the mind structures these varying impulses into familiar colors and shapes. There is no red in the "objective" universe, no blue or green—only fluctuations in the underlying non-material fields. Sensations of color—and all other such sensations—exist only in the mind.

In addition to such deceptive appearances, the effect of solidity is created by the negative electromagnetic charge of the electrons. If you push the north pole of one magnet toward the north pole of another, the two will appear to bounce off each other even before they touch. Like charges repel. Since every atom is surrounded by a pulsating wave of negative charge (which we refer to as one or more electrons), atoms ordinarily repel one another. Though they are mostly empty space, and totally non-material, the atoms are kept from interpenetrating by the electromagnetic force. When you bang your shin into a coffee table, the electromagnetic forces in your leg have been repelled by the electromagnetic forces in the table.

The world looks solid. It feels solid. But it's all an illusion. Sub-atomic "particles" are waves of no-thing-ness. At the most fundamental quantum mechanical level, the entire universe and your "physical" body are as insubstantial as the mind itself. Says physicist Paul Davies, "Many people have rejected scientific values because they regard materialism as a sterile and bleak philosophy, which reduces human beings to automatons and leaves no room for free will or creativity. These people can take heart: materialism is dead."[26]

THE MIND IN MATTER

At the subtlest level of inquiry, therefore, solid matter is no longer awkwardly interposed between human intelligence and nature's intelligence. Hard, inert lumps of stuff have only an apparent reality. Instead, at the finest sub-atomic levels, non-material waves dance in precise patterns. These non-material waves obey laws of nature that can be exactly modeled by mathematical formulas cognized in the human mind. In fact, the mathematical theory that describes the quantum behavior of the electromagnetic field is considered the most accurate and successful theory in the history of science.

In the insubstantial world of quantum mechanics, furthermore, the mind and nature have been found even more inextricably interwoven. Twentieth-century physicists have discovered to their astonishment that, at the sub-atomic level, observing a system *changes* the system.

This is not true in the macroscopic world around us. You can sit comfortably near a window and bird watch through binoculars without affecting either you or the bird. In quantum mechanical systems, however, to observe is to disturb. In their unobserved state, for example, electrons are in no particular place. Their position and momentum are described mathematically by probability waves. Probability wave functions do not give information about the precise location of an electron but about the mathematical odds for that position. At any given time, there will be a high probability of finding the electron in one or more areas, a lower probability of finding it in other areas, and a vanishingly small but still real probability of finding it absolutely anywhere in the universe.

When an actual observation is made, however, the electron is always found at some particular location. It leaves a spot on a photographic plate or a trail through a cloud chamber. The act of observation puts certain conditions or constraints on the system, forcing one particular resolution to emerge. A situation rich with possibility is collapsed to a single point value—what physicists call the collapse of the wave function—forever changing the original situation. What once had unbounded potential is now localized and specific. Says Eugene Wigner:

> . . . [T]he impression which one gains at an interaction, called also the result of an observation, modifies the wave function of the system. The modified wave function is, furthermore, in general unpredictable before the impression gained at the interaction has entered our consciousness: it is the entering of an impression into our consciousness which alters the wave function because it modifies our appraisal of the probabilities for different impressions which we expect to receive in the future. It is at this point that the consciousness enters the theory unavoidably and unalterably.[27]

In quantum mechanics, the mind of the scientist has thus become intermingled with the object being studied. The subjective and the objective can no longer be separated. In the words of Niels Bohr, who took the lead in development of quantum theories in the 1930s, ". . . we are both spectators and actors in the great drama of existence."[28] Physicist John Wheeler, who made his reputation in the second half of this century with research on black holes, expresses the same idea more pointedly. If the observer changes what he observes, Wheeler says, this

> . . . destroys the concept of the world 'sitting out there' with the observer safely separated from it by a 20 centimeter slab of glass. . . .

The universe will never afterward be the same. To describe what has happened one has to cross out that old word 'observer' and put in its place the new word 'participator.' In some strange sense, the universe is a participatory universe.[29]

As the French physicist Bernard d'Espagnat commented in an article in *Scientific American*: "The doctrine that the world is made up of objects whose existence is independent of human consciousness turns out to be in conflict with quantum mechanics and with the facts established by experiment."[30]

Nineteenth-century physics may have attempted to argue consciousness out of existence, but twentieth-century physics has rescued it from scientific purgatory. In the twentieth century, objective investigation has rediscovered the subjective role in the physical world. Says Wigner:

> When the province of physical theory was extended to encompass microscopic phenomena, through the creation of quantum mechanics, the concept of consciousness came to the fore again: it was not possible to formulate the laws of quantum mechanics in a fully consistent way without reference to the consciousness. . . . It will remain remarkable, in whatever way our future concepts may develop, that the very study of the external world led to the conclusion that the content of the consciousness is an ultimate reality.[31]

CONSCIOUSNESS AT THE BASIS

These discoveries have been a shock to common sense notions about nature and human nature. Solid, inert substance has disappeared from the scientific view of the world. Intelligence and consciousness, on the other hand, are found even at the deepest levels of nature's functioning. For such reasons, in the view of many of this century's leading physicists, the most fundamental aspect of nature is not matter but mind. Max Planck, who was the first pioneer in the development of quantum theory, expressed his view forcibly: "I regard consciousness as fundamental. I regard matter as derivative from consciousness."[32] Exploring the implications of the new quantum physics, Sir James Jeans said,

> Today there is a wide measure of agreement, which on the physical side of science approaches almost to unanimity, that the stream of knowledge is heading toward a non-mechanical reality; the universe begins to look more like a great thought than a great machine.[33]

Expanding the logic behind this conclusion, Jeans said,

> . . . the old dualism of mind and matter . . . seems likely to disappear, not through matter becoming in any way more shadowy or insubstantial than heretofore, or through mind becoming resolved into a function of the working of matter, but through substantial matter resolving itself into a creation and manifestation of mind.[34]

Sir Arthur Eddington is the physicist whose experiments first confirmed Einstein's theory of relativity; he was also one of the most thoughtful and penetrating philosophers in the field of physics. On this topic he has said:

> All through the physical world runs that unknown *content* which must surely be the stuff of our own consciousness. . . . [W]e have found that where science has progressed the farthest, the mind has regained from nature that which the mind has put into nature. We have found a strange footprint on the shores of the unknown. We have devised profound theories, one after another to account for its origin. At last, we have succeeded in reconstructing the creature that made the footprint. And lo! it is our own.[35]

Elsewhere, Eddington gave perhaps the best short summation of the idea that consciousness and creation are one and the same: ". . . the stuff of the world is mind-stuff."[36]

THE ACCURACY OF SUBJECTIVE KNOWLEDGE

If consciousness is primary, if physical reality is created from pure intelligence, if world-stuff is mind-stuff—then the progress of objective, scientific investigation has arrived at the Vedic understanding attained through subjective, inward investigation. Intelligence is the basis of existence. Subjectivity is the basis of objectivity.

Moreover, it would appear that this subjective understanding of nature can only be validated through subjective investigation. The objective approach—logic and experiment—cannot be definitive, because logic and experiment by themselves have strict limitations. As philosophers of science point out, it is not actually possible to prove something true through logic and experiment. There are two types of logic, for example, deductive and inductive, and neither is self-sufficient. Deductive logic can be rigorous, but it starts with premises which are themselves outside of logic. "All roads lead to Rome; this is a road; this road leads to Rome." The deduction from the premise is faultless, but the premise itself is simply given. The premise cannot be proven within the system; that is, it can't be proven by deduction from itself. You can't lift yourself by your own bootstraps.

Inductive logic, on the other hand, which is the basis of experiment, is likewise incomplete. You gather facts one after another until you see where they are headed. If you drop a stone 50 times and it falls to the ground every time, you assume that dropped stones always fall. This is sensible, but not certain. The next stone could rise. Inductive logic is an educated guess.

For these reasons, the philosophy of science indicates that you can't prove anything through scientific investigation. You can only disprove. Experiments can show your premise false (you can find a road that doesn't lead to Rome), but not true (no matter how many roads have led to Rome, the next one might not). A theory is considered scientific if it is logically consistent, open to disproof (or falsification), and experimentation does not disprove it.

In any search for truth, therefore, objective scientific investigation is admittedly incomplete. As Paul Davies says,

We are barred from ultimate knowledge, from ultimate explanation, by the very rules of reasoning that prompt us to seek such an explanation in the first place. If we wish to progress beyond, we have to embrace a different concept of 'understanding' from that of rational explanation.[37]

Such a different concept of understanding is provided by direct, subjective intuition. Moreover, by combining subjective and objective approaches, we then have the makings of a complete system of investigation. Subjective intuition (cognition, revelation) could provide new premises. Logic and experiment could attempt to disprove them.

This second step would still be important, of course. Even if we formally admit intuition as a valid means for obtaining knowledge, rational investigation would still be necessary. An inner, subjective experience can be wholly inaccurate; pink elephants are more likely the result of inebriants than intuition. A cloudy mind yields cloudy ideas.

On the other hand, failures by cloudy minds do not invalidate discoveries by those with clearer awareness. Recall that, within the elegant intellects possessed by great scientists, deep and sudden intuitions often bring a sense of certainty with them, as if they have been read from Erdös' book. When a refined awareness truly sees a subtle reality deep within its own nature, logic and experiment seem but formal exercise. Einstein was once asked what he would think if an experiment disproved his theory of relativity. "So much the worse for the experiment," he said. "The theory is right."[38]

To such people, inner, intuitive knowledge seems more certain than logic or experiment. But is this possible? Can the mind itself yield more certainty than objective investigation? It's a topic that has been rigorously investigated.

The mathematician Kurt Gödel discovered his paradigm-altering incompleteness theorem while systematically questioning whether any logical system can verify its own premises. The answer to the main question was no, and in the process Gödel discovered something more startling. Within every logical system, Gödel found, there is at least one true statement which the system itself can't prove to be true. His investigations were mathematical, but one of the mysteriously true statements he discovered can be translated roughly into English as, "You can't prove this statement is true." The truth of the statement is, as it says in the Declaration of Independence, self-evident. If you could prove the statement true, that would make it false. Therefore, you can see that it's true that you can't prove it's true. So it is true, but unprovable. This discovery showed, first, that any logical system is incomplete—incapable of accounting for all truth. Second, it showed that the mind can recognize an absolute truth independent of logic and experiment. The mind can do within itself what logic and experiment cannot do: produce complete certainty.

This experience of complete certainty accompanies every profound cognition. The mind "sees" the truth, direct and unaided. Intelligence cognizes its own fluctuations firsthand—rather than recognizing (re-cognizing) truth secondhand, through an intermediary such as logic or experiment.

TRAINING FOR SUBJECTIVE INVESTIGATION

This discovery places a premium on the refined mind. The more subtle and penetrating the awareness, the more profound the discoveries it can theoretically make. The goal of such a refined awareness, moreover, is to know itself—to experience the finest and most fundamental fluctuations of its own nature. Discoveries about nature's intelligence are made within human intelligence. Discoveries about the outer, objective world are made deep within one's own intelligence, at the source of subjectivity.

All of this raises a practical question. Can we do anything to enhance this ability of subjective investigation? To do better experiments, physicists build larger and larger particle accelerators. But such machinery is for objective investigation. You can't use a machine to enhance subjective investigation, the mind's inner ability to experience its own nature. In the tradition of Western science, there is no record of systematic and effective techniques to enhance intuition. Gödel used informal forms of meditation such as lying down and deliberately ignoring sense impressions. Princeton's Ed Witten, perhaps the most influential mathematical physicist now working on superunified field theories (the "theory of everything"), does some of his best work lying in a hammock. Such approaches have been so unreliable, however, that the true inner revelation is not common. Commenting on this relative dearth of inner revelation, physicist Fred Hoyle reported on a conversation he had with fellow-physicist Richard Feynman:

> Some years ago I had a graphic description from Dick Feynman of what a moment of inspiration feels like, and of it being followed by an enormous sense of euphoria, lasting for maybe two or three days. I asked how often had it happened, to which Feynman replied 'four', at which we both agreed that twelve days of euphoria was not a great reward for a lifetime's work.[39]

The Western scientific tradition appears to offer no path to perfect the human mechanism for discovery. The ancient Vedic tradition, however, did not leave the intuitive experience to chance. Rather, the Vedic tradition has always been based on a series of systematic techniques intended to unfold the full potential of human consciousness. If the mind is a direct route to accurate information, then the mind's ability to perceive its own finest fluctuations should be deliberately cultivated. This is the role of meditation.

Medical investigators may think of the Transcendental Meditation technique as primarily a relaxation technique. They may view it as a means to avoid the free radical attacks caused by stress and tension. But from the standpoint of Maharishi Ayur-Ved, the Transcendental Meditation technique has a much more profound role. It is intended to refine human awareness. It is a technique to enhance subjective investigation, by allowing the mind to experience its own deepest level. The Vedic tradition has supplied systematic meditation techniques to allow our inner eye to adjust to the deeper levels of intelligence within the mind.

As Maharishi himself has made clear, this does not mean that all people who hone their awareness with regular meditation will go out for a Sunday walk and cognize the theory of relativity. Different people have different natural tendencies, from science to gardening, from business to art to parenting. Maharishi does indicate, however, that regular experience of the deepest levels of intelligence within the mind brings each individual more closely in tune with the deepest levels of intelligence in nature. What physicists have barely glimpsed, he reports with confidence: Human intelligence and nature's intelligence are one and the same. By coming into accord with one's own inner intelligence, one comes into accord with the intelligence expressed in the laws of nature.

MODERN SCIENCE AND VEDIC SCIENCE

We set out in this chapter to discover how ayurvedic vaidyas could have found highly effective health modalities without the aid of objective scientific investigation. We set out, specifically, to understand how Bharadwaja was able to use subjective technologies of consciousness to directly cognize, deep within his own awareness, accurate information about the physical body. Though this sounds superficially unscientific, it turns out that objective researchers also make use of sudden subjective intuitions. These subjective intuitions are often precisely accurate. Scientists have explained this accuracy by postulating that (1) the human mind has direct access to a realm of pure intelligence and (2) the subtle impulses experienced in this realm by mathematically trained minds yield mathematical structures that precisely describe laws of nature in the physical world. Thus, the Western scientific tradition indicates that it is possible to instantly cognize fundamental truths about the physical world; great scientists have done it repeatedly.

We have also heard the reasoning that has led many leading physicists to give a theoretical understanding for this phenomenon. They have concluded that the entire physical world is, in fact, based on pure intelligence or pure consciousness. In this view, what appears superficially as the physical world is actually a matrix of fluctuations in an unbounded field of consciousness. Why can laws of nature be experienced in human intelligence? Because these laws themselves are nothing but waves, or fluctuations, in an underlying field of intelligence— intelligence continuous with the human mind. Researchers who are sufficiently "awake" can directly intuit or cognize truths about the physical world; in cognizing the finest impulses of their own minds, they cognize the finest impulses that govern the outer world.

This gives us a way to understand Bharadwaja's experience. The range and detail of his cognitions—much more extensive than typical intuitions by modern scientists—we can only ascribe to his many years of practice of meditation techniques, and to the enlivenment of the underlying field of consciousness created by the scores of Vedic sages meditating with him. In modern science, direct, subjective investigation has been haphazard, usually unsought and often unknown. In the Vedic tradition, it has been the result of systematic preparation and specific technique.

The concepts discussed in this chapter may shed light on more than Bharadwaja's cognitions. If, as Jeans said, substantial matter has resolved itself into a manifestation of mind; if, as Eddington said, the unknown content of the material world is consciousness—then it would appear that our theories of medicine are in need of revision. The mechanistic, purely material view of the body is based on outmoded, nineteenthcentury theories. Physicists discarded these theories long ago. Now it appears that medical science must catch up. If the

body has its basis in intelligence, then medicine must understand and address this underlying, non-material reality.

It is time to discuss a consciousness paradigm of physical
health.

Notes

1. Quoted in Hadamard J, An Essay on *The Psychology of Invention in the Mathematical Field* (Princeton University Press, Princeton, 1949), p. 12

2. Hoyle F, *Univ Cardiff Rep* 70(1981): 43

3. Penrose R, *The Emperor's New Mind: Concerning Computers, Minds, and the Laws of Physics* (Oxford University Press, Oxford, 1989), p. 420

4. Asimov I, *The Left Hand of the Electron* (Dell Publishing Co. Inc., New York, 1974), pp. 196-8

5. Littlewood JE, *Rockefeller Univ Rev* (September-October)(1967): 112-8

6. Hadamard, *Psychology* (see note 1), p. 13

7. Asimov, *The Left* (see note 4), pp. 191-2

8. Penrose, *Emperor's* (see note 3), p. 428

9. Rucker R, *Infinity and the Mind* (Birkhauser, Boston, 1982), p. 36

10. Quoted in Barrow JD, *Pi in the Sky: Counting, Thinking, and Being* (Clarendon Press, Oxford, 1992), pp. 279-80

11. Davies P, *The Mind of God: The Scientific Basis for a Rational World* (Simon & Schuster, New York, 1992), p. 154

12. Quoted in Barrow, *Pi* (see note 10), p. 278

13. Davies, *Mind* (see note 11), p. 140

14. Jeans J, *The Mysterious Universe* (Cambridge University Press, Cambridge, 1930), p. 132

15. Davies P, *Superforce: The Search for a Grand Unified Theory of Nature* (Touchstone, Simon & Schuster, New York, 1984), p. 51

16. Jeans, *Mysterious* (see note 14), p. 130

17. Wigner E, *Communic Pure Appl Mathem* 13(1960): 1

18. Davies, *Mind* (see note 11), p. 148

19. Penrose, *Emperor's* (see note 3), pp. 430

20. Weyl H, *Mind and Nature* (University of Pennsylvania Press, Philadelphia, 1934), p. 36

21. Quoted in Augros RM, Stanciu GN, *The New Story of Science: Mind and the Universe* (Regnery Gateway, Inc., Lake Bluff, 1984), p. 167-8

22. Wigner E, "Remarks on the Mind-Body Question" in *The Scientist Speculates*, Good IJ, ed. (William Heinemann, Ltd., London, 1961), first page

23. Capra F, *The Tao of Physics: An Explanation of the Parallels Between Modern Physics and Eastern Mysticism* (Shambhala, Boston, 1991), p. 210

24. Davies, *Superforce* (see note 15), p. 41

25. Quoted in Capek M, *The Philosophical Impact of Contemporary Physics* (Van Nostrand, Princeton, 1961), p. 319

26. Davies P, *The Matter Myth: Dramatic Discoveries That Challenge Our Understanding of Physical Reality* (Simon & Schuster, New York, 1992), p. 13

27. Wigner, "Remarks" (see note 22), third page

28. Quoted in Weyl, *Mind* (see note 20), p. 100

29. Quoted in Oates RM Jr., *Creating Heaven on Earth* (Heaven on Earth Publications, Fairfield, 1990), p. 132

30. d'Espagnat B, *Scientific American* 241(5)(1979): 158-81

31. Wigner, "Remarks" (see note 22), second page

32. Klein DB, *The Concept of Consciousness: A Survey* (University of Nebraska Press, Lincoln, 1984), quoted in front matter

33. Jeans, *Mysterious* (see note 14), p. 148

34. Ibid, pp. 148-9

35. Eddington A, *Space, Time and Gravitation: An Outline of the General Relativity Theory* (Harper & Row, New York, 1959), pp. 200-1

36. Eddington A, *The Nature of the Physical World* (The University of Michigan Press, Ann Arbor, 1974), p. 276

37. Davies, *Mind* (see note 11), p. 231

38. Ibid, p. 175-6

39. Hoyle, *Univ* (see note 2), p. 42

From Mind to Body

Pasteur discovered microbes. Molecular biologists then looked more deeply and found free radicals. In the last chapter, we went deeper still, past molecules and atoms and sub-atomic particles, to the unbounded, non-material field at the basis of creation. It is encouraging to speculate that this fundamental, field-level standpoint can give us leverage on free radicals.

If you can operate at the level of water, you can control the waves. If you can operate at the level of the quantum mechanical field—where apparently solid matter has dissolved and only the intelligence of the laws of nature is lively—perhaps you can influence the waves or fluctuations which make up our sub-atomic particles and atoms, our molecules and cells.

There is only one system of medicine I know which takes such a field-level approach. There is only one which bases a comprehensive set of practical approaches on the most fundamental level of intelligence in nature. It is the ancient ayurvedic system of India—now revived as Maharishi Ayur-Ved.

THE REVIVAL OF KNOWLEDGE

A systematic revival of this knowledge was necessary because, in recent centuries, ayurveda had become fragmented and unreliable. During centuries of colonial rule in India, ayurvedic institutions were not officially supported and often, in fact, were suppressed. Much important clinical and theoretical knowledge was lost. Experts in the various approaches of ayurveda—specialists in herbal medicines, purification procedures, pulse diagnosis, and many other modalities—lost contact with each other and even began to compete with one another. Most significantly, the central role of consciousness, of meditation and other mental techniques, was temporarily eclipsed.

When Maharishi Mahesh Yogi turned his attention to ayurveda in the 1980s, his stated goal was to revive the system in its comprehensive and integrated form—with the help of leading vaidyas of our time, and in accordance with the classical texts. Most especially, his intent was to restore the role of consciousness to its central position—both theoretically and through practical techniques.

In one sense, it is no surprise that this restoration of ayurveda in our time has been undertaken by a maharishi (the word means "great seer"). In the *Charak Samhita*, such leadership is said to be the usual situation: "Ayurved, the science of life, has been taught by the maharishis who are devoted to righteousness (*dharma*) and the welfare of the people, and not their own earnings and enjoyment."[1] Maharishi's 35 years of work to bring Vedic knowledge around the world have provided evidence of his devotion to "righteousness and the welfare of the people," and now in Maharishi Ayur-Ved, there is once again a prevention-oriented system of natural health care that has its basis in consciousness.

A CONSCIOUSNESS PARADIGM

In much of this book, we have focused on the minute building blocks of the physical world. We have focused especially on rogue molecules, on free radicals: how they are created, how they cause disease, how they can be controlled. Our larger concern has been physical health: how to improve the health of the individual and society, how to reduce suffering and increase life span, how to resolve the health care crisis in America and around the world. But the last chapter took a turn toward the non-material. It indicated that the human body is based in a field of pure intelligence, or pure consciousness. How does such a new, consciousness-based paradigm relate to the free radical challenge?

One answer can be stated briefly. The free radical paradigm has at last provided for Western medicine a unified theory of disease. It has provided a single molecular mechanism that can account for much of illness and aging. What this seems to demand is a single, unified theory of medicine.

The allopathic approach does not provide such an integrated outlook. In fact, the allopathic approach is deliberately *ad hoc*. It goes disease by disease, feeling its way through experimentation toward specific cures for specific maladies. There is no conception of a single, underlying theory of medical practice.

The latest discoveries of modern physics, however, have paved the way for such a comprehensive theory—a theory that includes both body and mind. Perhaps a system of medicine based on consciousness can offer a field-level framework for a unified and holistic approach to control free radicals and produce ideal health.

To explore this hypothesis, we must first understand much more about consciousness—and its relation to the physical world. We must master the consciousness paradigm in much greater detail. We need to understand how consciousness can give rise to matter. Specifically, we need to understand how consciousness can give rise to the physical body. Most practically, we need to know how to make use of such knowledge. We need to know how to intervene when the mind-to-body process has gone awry, how to restore health to a body diseased.

AN EXPERT IN CONSCIOUSNESS

In the last chapter, we turned to experts in objective science. Now we want to explore a subjective approach to life and health. For this, the expert with whom I am most familiar is Maharishi Mahesh Yogi, the founder of Maharishi Ayur-Ved (Maharishi can be pronounced Mah-hah-REE-shi or Mah-HAR-shi; Ved rhymes with *wade*: EYE-yur VADE). Because he has devoted 35 years to bringing the ancient Vedic knowledge to the whole world, and to integrating that knowledge with the best of Western science, Maharishi is widely considered today's leading exponent of consciousness-based theories and technologies. As I have become more familiar with his achievements, I have gained increasing confidence in his expertise:

• Maharishi is the first teacher in the Vedic tradition to have systematized the teaching of meditation, allowing him to train thousands of other people to give instruction in Transcendental Meditation.

• He is the first exponent of the Vedic knowledge to have encouraged objective research on subjective meditation techniques, and the first to have seen a large outpouring of studies. Rather than pitting subjective and objective approaches against one another, he has led a unification of the two that he calls Vedic Science.

• After 20 years of scientific investigation, Maharishi has seen the combined research clearly indicate that the mental and physical approaches he advocates are much more effective than any others yet tested scientifically. His expertise has been validated objectively.

• He is the first teacher in the Vedic tradition who has worked extensively to detail the mechanics of intelligence—in nature and in the human mind—and to align these understandings with the most profound discoveries of scientific theory. He is also the first, on this basis, to found universities (such as Maharishi International University in the United States and Maharishi Vedic Universities in many countries around the world) which teach all disciplines in the light of this integrated understanding of life.

CONSCIOUSNESS IS PRIMARY

When Maharishi talks of consciousness, when he discusses the relationship between consciousness and the material world, he begins his analysis where modern physics has left off. He asserts definitely that the basis of the physical universe—and the physical body—is an unbounded field of pure intelligence, or pure consciousness. All waves are fluctuations in the unbounded ocean. In the same way, he maintains that all the forces and "particles" of nature are fluctuations in an "unbounded ocean of consciousness."

We have seen that leading physicists have glimpsed this "unknown content" of physical reality. But through experimental science, this subjective basis of nature can only be surmised, not proven. Quantum mechanical physics has penetrated to the level of unbounded, omnipresent fields—fields which are both non-material and lively with mathematically describable intelligence. At this level, solid matter has disappeared. And where solid objects cease, "object-ive" science has been left behind. As we have seen, moreover, many scientists feel that consciousness—pure subjectivity—must now be included in physics. Maharishi has commented on this transition:

> Progress depends on new discoveries; the objective approach of modern science . . . has invited modern science to transcend the objective approach and design new theories of consciousness and a new experimental approach using the subjective approach . . . . Now, if progress is to continue, research has to be in the field of pure subjectivity and the approach has to be subjective.[2]

Maharishi mentions another reason for the importance of a subjective approach. He points out that modern science, being objective, brings only intellectual understanding about the laws of nature. The physicist may understand the law of gravity or the law of least action. But this intellectual understanding, he says, "does not penetrate into the life of the scientist."[3] Despite profound intellectual knowledge about the sub-atomic basis of nature, for example, physicists are no better equipped to live a long, healthy, and fulfilling life than anyone else. Factual information about nature does not change their physiological functioning, their emotional life, or their career performance. Maharishi says of such a scientist, "He can do some little jugglery here and there in the field of creation, converting this into that and that into this, but he himself is open to all kinds of destructive values because the modern approach to the investigation of natural law does not and cannot enable the scientist to imbibe knowledge and live it in daily life."[4]

This does not mean that Maharishi scorns objective science. In his Vedic Science, objective investigation still provides external validation for truths first gained internally, in consciousness. But objective investigation is no longer understood as separate and self-sufficient. In keeping with many of the scientists we have quoted so far, he feels that, "Now is the time for scientists to investigate into the total reality of life without excluding consciousness. Today, those who exclude consciousness are not with the times, they are far behind."[5]

FROM MIND TO MATTER

The central question concerns the relationship between consciousness and the physical world, between mind and body. How does a non-material field of pure consciousness give rise to the apparently solid world we live in? According to Maharishi, the question is answered by the very nature of consciousness. It is *conscious*. It is aware. And if, at the basis of creation, consciousness is the sole reality, then it has only itself to be aware of. Because of its own nature, Maharishi maintains that pure consciousness "cannot hold itself back" from knowing itself; it is therefore "completely self-referral"—aware of itself alone.

Thus, the very nature of consciousness ensures that an undifferentiated unity—pure consciousness—automatically becomes a tri-partite diversity. As consciousness knows itself, it becomes knower, process of knowing, and known—or observer, process of observation, and observed. Consciousness is the subject, the object, and the connection between the two.

From one standpoint, therefore, pure consciousness is solitary, it is unity. From another, it is manifold, it is diversity.

In the field of pure consciousness, Maharishi states, these standpoints alternate back and forth with infinite frequency. This rapid alternation imparts an infinite dynamism to a field otherwise absolutely silent. Maharishi explains that,

> The three-in-one structure of pure knowledge is a kind of pulsating reality—from unity to three, from three to unity. In this pulsating unity, this range of activity—back and forth, expansion and contraction—we find [the basis] of life.[6]

In Sanskrit, the language of the Vedic tradition, the knower is termed *Rishi*, the process of knowing *Devata*, and the object of knowing *Chhandas*. The unity of the three is termed *Samhita* (unitedness, collectedness). Samhita stands for the togetherness, or the unified state—the state of perfect balance—of Rishi, Devata, and Chhandas, which interact dynamically.

THE VARIETY OF CREATION

In Maharishi's understanding, this is where the variety of creation begins. The unity or singularity of pure consciousness spontaneously "breaks" into diversity, the silence of pure consciousness into dynamism.

Furthermore, once it has begun, this internal, self-referral process of elaboration continues indefinitely. When consciousness becomes aware of itself, the knower becomes aware of the known, the Rishi becomes aware of Chhandas. This changes the situation. The knower, or Rishi, is no longer simple, but is colored by awareness of the known, or Chhandas. This more complex Rishi also becomes aware of the Chhandas, changing the situation further. In a stepwise progression, the original three—knower, process of knowing, and known—interact an infinite number of times, assuming infinite degrees of shadings and complexities. Eventually, this process of self-referral becomes so rich with complexity that the original unity, or Samhita, is hidden from view.

People often go to movies to forget themselves, to get caught up in the action on the screen and temporarily ignore their own lives. Maharishi explains that, in a similar way, the Rishi, or knower, gets caught up in the complexity of knowing and known. It forgets the silent, unified state of Samhita, and only diversity appears to remain. What was once pure consciousness alone has become an experience of infinite variety. And this variety, Maharishi indicates, is the world we see:

> The self-referral state of consciousness is that one element in nature on the ground of which the infinite variety of creation is continuously emerging, growing, and dissolving. The whole field of change emerges from this field of non-change, from this self-referral, immortal state of consciousness.[7]

Maharishi describes the silent state of Samhita as unmanifest, absolute, and transcendental (beyond all activity and change). The "field of change" emerges from the interaction of knower, process of knowing, and known. Maharishi describes this ever-changing state as dynamic, manifest, and relative (the knower, for example, has meaning only relative to the known). He indicates that the constant alternation of the silence of Samhita with the dynamic interplay of Rishi, Devata, and Chhandas is the basis of the physical universe:

That self-referral activity cannot be hampered from outside. It is the most basic performance in nature. It transcends all activity of natural law in the relative field, but yet is always lively as the basis of the classical, physical world. It is the most refined level of quantum-mechanical activity of nature, from where absolute orderliness controls, commands, and governs all affairs of the universe.[8]

These interactions at the basis of the physical world explain how, in the words of Sir James Jeans, matter can be "a creation and manifestation of mind." We have seen in the last chapter that solid matter has no real existence. The universe is made of waves, or fluctuations, or vibrations, in the underlying non-material field of pure consciousness. Maharishi maintains that these fluctuations are stirred up by the self-referral mechanics of consciousness as it knows itself. The entire universe results from consciousness interacting within itself. The sequentially elaborating interactions between Rishi, Devata, and Chhandas, Maharishi indicates, are ". . . those fine creative impulses that are engaged in transforming the field of intelligence into the field of matter."[9]

THE INTELLIGENCE OF DNA

In the physical body, this sequential unfoldment of intelligence into matter can be seen taking place at a relatively advanced stage. The DNA molecule encodes all the intelligence that forms the entire physiology. A code is a pattern; in fact, in one sense, all intelligence is pattern. In the DNA, the pattern is made of specific sequences of four nucleotide base molecules. It is not these molecules that are intelligent, but rather the unmanifest, non-material pattern in which those molecules are arranged; the four nucleotides only show what the pattern is, as leaves floating on a stream show where the currents flow. It is, in fact, true that the nucleotide base molecules come and go constantly, replacing one another as place holders in the underlying pattern.

This intelligent pattern embodied in the DNA itself remains unchanging and uninvolved, but it gives rise to the physiology in steps of sequential progression. As Maharishi says, "This is the creative process—intelligence converting itself into matter. . . . DNA starts the process with an impulse of information. RNA carries it, and then the proteins arise. Here is conversion of intelligence, or consciousness, into matter."[10]

Just as the DNA remains unchanged and uninvolved while its intelligence elaborates into the entire body, the unified field of pure consciousness remains uninvolved as it elaborates into the physical universe. In Maharishi's words,

> The self-referral intelligence at the unmanifest basis of creation remains uninvolved in the creative process, but the creative process owes its emergence and draws its vitality from that self-referral performance of pure intelligence. The self-referral state of pure consciousness, while remaining uninvolved with the creative process in nature, is an infinitely dynamic, inexhaustible source of energy and creativity. On that basis the whole creation goes on perpetually in its infinite variety, multiplying itself all the time.[11]

THE UNIFIED FIELD OF NATURAL LAW

To be more than abstract theory, such ideas must generate practical results. Investigation of the electromagnetic field, for example, has already led to lasers and holograms. Theory produces technology. If the self-interacting mechanics of consciousness create the physical body, knowledge of this process should also give rise to practical technologies.

In the next chapter we will review the many technologies of Maharishi Ayur-Ved. Before we consider them, however, we can usefully cast one more glance at the field of physics. Maharishi frequently refers to the field of pure consciousness—the collectedness of observer, observation, and observed—as the "unified field of intelligence," the "unified field of nature's intelligence," or the "unified field of natural law."

This understanding of nature's fundamental unity has recently been paralleled by the latest discoveries in modern quantum mechanical physics.

Albert Einstein was deeply convinced that the laws of nature had a simple, unified foundation. He spent the last half of his life working to demonstrate this underlying unity. Unfortunately, the theoretical tools and understanding needed to achieve such a unification were not available in Einstein's lifetime.

Within the past 20 years, however, a number of significant breakthroughs have led to the development of completely unified theories. All the apparently distinct force and matter fields that structure creation are now understood simply as differing modes of excitation of one underlying field. A single guitar string can be made to vibrate in many ways, providing a wide variety of notes. In the same way, *superunified* quantum field theories say that all of nature results from differing vibrations of a single unified field—also known as the super-field, or superstring field.

Although this project of superunification is not yet complete, progress to date has yielded a number of meaningful insights—parallels with the theoretical picture put forth in Maharishi's Vedic Science. The leading expert in these parallels is theoretical physicist John Hagelin. Harvard-trained, Dr. Hagelin has been mentioned in the national media as a possible Nobel laureate for his work on unified field theories. After working at the European Center for Nuclear Research and the Stanford Linear Accelerator, Dr. Hagelin is now a Professor of Physics at Maharishi International University and Director of MIU's Institute of Science, Technology and Public Policy. His ongoing work in physics is supported by grants from the National Science Foundation.

Intelligence of natural law: In academic articles and lectures delivered at universities and research centers worldwide,

Dr. Hagelin has focused on several aspects of the unified field. In the first place, he points out that the deepest levels of nature display the most concentrated intelligence:

> As the laws of nature become more compact and concentrated, intelligence can be said to become more concentrated. If, as particle theorists are inclined to believe, all the laws of nature have their ultimate origin in the dynamics of the unified field, then the unified field must itself embody the total intelligence of nature's functioning.[12]

Silence and dynamism: Second, Maharishi describes the unified field of intelligence as both silent and infinitely dynamic. Dr. Hagelin points out that every quantum field, including the unified field, has an identical dual nature. As we have seen, particles and forces are nothing but waves in these underlying fields. When these waves quiet down completely and there are, thus, *no* particles or forces, the field is said to be in its *state of least excitation.* Because of the absence of particles and forces this is also known as the *vacuum state.*

This would seem to be a state of complete inertia, but in fact the opposite is true. The state of least excitation is not really a vacuum. It is not flat and inert. Instead, this state of seeming silence results from infinite dynamism. The field actually teems with an infinite variety of waves and fluctuations. The illusion of inertia is created because all these waves cancel each other out. With infinite waves available, the peak of any wave is always exactly canceled by the trough of another. In Dr. Hagelin's phrase, "the state of least excitation results from the simultaneous superposition of all possible shapes of the field." As Maharishi says of the unified field of intelligence, silence coexists with dynamism.

Three in one: Third, Dr. Hagelin has shown that the unified field has a 3-in-1 structure. Mathematical descriptions of the field show that the Bose fields (the basic force fields of nature) and Fermi fields (the basic matter fields) are connected and unified by the dynamical principle of gauge super-symmetry. "From this perspective," Dr. Hagelin says, "the unified field or superfield corresponds to the Samhita of Maharishi's Vedic Science."[13]

Self-interacting: In addition, Dr. Hagelin shows that the unified field works through self-interacting mechanics. There is nothing "outside" the unified field. The various subtle aspects of the unified field interact together, providing the dynamism which appears as varying fluctuations and vibrations of the field. These various fluctuations of the field create our world—they become the more superficial and apparently disunited force and matter fields that structure nature.

Moreover, these transitions occur as a process of, in Dr. Hagelin's words, "spontaneous, sequential, dynamical symmetry breaking." The perfect balance, or supersymmetry, within the unified field spontaneously breaks, and a sequence of less perfectly balanced states emerges. The end result is the universe we see. As Dr. Hagelin points out, these subtle internal dynamics of creation, as understood by the latest quantum mechanical theories, are far from any understanding of nature put forward previously in the age of science. They are, however, markedly parallel with the understandings Maharishi discusses in his Vedic Science.

Objectivity and subjectivity: Finally, Dr. Hagelin indicates that the very concept of a unified field implies that the objective and subjective worlds must come together. The whole history of science has revealed a march toward increasing unity. Electricity and magnetism, for example, were once considered separate and distinct. But 19th-century experiments showed them to be two aspects of the single electromagnetic force. Now, superunified theories have defined one unified field of *all* force and matter fields. The last step of unification is to include not only the force and matter fields of the objective world, but also consciousness. Dr. Hagelin says,

> Most particle theorists would agree that the unified field is the source of both subjective and objective existence. This is because most physicists would like to avoid the necessity of introducing anything external to the laws of physics, such as a metaphysical explanation for consciousness, feeling that the unified field should be the dynamical origin of all phenomena.[14]

Dr. Hagelin also remarks that in the unified field, there is no room for disunion. There is no formal way to describe subjectivity as distinct from objectivity. This explains why, at the quantum mechanical level of nature, the observer changes the observed. The two are in fact indissolubly linked. In Dr. Hagelin's words,

> Since it is generally assumed that the unified field is the only dynamical degree of freedom present at the superunified scale, to the extent that a subject-object relationship can be defined there at all, the 'observer' and the 'observed' must both be found within the dynamical self-interaction of the unified field itself. From this perspective, the unified field is formally as much a field of subjectivity as a field of objectivity. Hence the proposed identity between the 'objective' unified field of modern theoretical physics and a 'subjective' unified field of consciousness is consistent from a logical standpoint.[15]

THE CONSTITUTION OF THE UNIVERSE

It is not only the field of physics that produces parallels with the unified field of pure consciousness. Because this unified field is the source of all the laws of nature, Maharishi has also called it the "Constitution of the Universe." The constitution of any nation is the basis of all the man-made laws in that nation; in the same way, the Constitution of the Universe is the basis of all the natural laws in the universe.

This Constitution has a literal reality; it can actually be written out. The unified field of physics is described in a complex sequence of mathematical equations known as the *Lagrangian*. This mathematical code describes the internal mechanics within the unified field which give rise to all the other force and matter fields, and thus to the entire universe.

In the ancient Vedic literature, according to Maharishi, there is also a precise description of the unified field. This is Rik Ved, the fountainhead of all the Vedic literature. In Maharishi's Vedic Science, the true content of Rik Ved is not given by translating words and gaining intellectual meaning. Instead, Rik Ved itself can be thought of as a code for, or embodiment of, the laws of nature in their most fundamental form. The sound of each syllable, the precise sequence of the syllables, and the mathematical relationships between the syllables, phrases, lines, verses, and stanzas all characterize the laws of nature and their interactions—just as the mathematical formulas of the Lagrangian do. In fact, Maharishi has worked with Dr. Hagelin to bring out precise parallels between the mathematical structure of the knowledge in Rik Ved and the mathematical structure in the Lagrangian.

Work on such parallels with DNA has also begun. The DNA represents the intelligence of nature as it is expressed in the physiology. In a sense, the DNA is the constitution of the physical body—the basis of all the laws of nature that uphold the body's structure and activity. In Maharishi's understanding, this intelligence (or knowledge) embodied in the DNA reflects the intelligence in the Constitution of the Universe. The structure of the DNA therefore matches the structure of Rik Ved. An example can make the principle clear.

Rik Ved: Maharishi explains that all the knowledge in Rik Ved develops in a sequential unfoldment that is completely orderly and mathematical in structure. First, the totality of knowledge is embodied in compactified form in the first syllable of Rik Ved. This concentrated knowledge is then elaborated by the sequential progression of the 24 syllables in the first line. The complete knowledge available in the first line, in turn, is elaborated further in the next eight lines of the first sukt (stanza). These eight lines consist of 24 padas (phrases) of 8 syllables each, comprising 8 x 24 = 192 syllables altogether. Ultimately, in subsequent stages of unfoldment, these 192 syllables of the first sukt get elaborated in the 192 suktas that comprise the first mandal (circular, cyclical, eternal structure) of the Rik Ved, which in turn gives rise to the rest of the Ved and the entire Vedic literature. Thus, at important stages in the elaboration, complete knowledge is encoded in structures containing 192 units.

DNA: The DNA code is represented by the sequence of four different nucleotide base "letters" as they join into three-letter "words" known as codons. The DNA molecule therefore contains 64 different codons (four different nucleotides, with only three taken at a time, in every possible arrangement, yield 64 different possible arrangements). Since each of the 64 codons has three nucleotides, there are 3 x 64 = 192 nucleotide bases involved altogether.

Moreover, the three nucleotides in each codon can be seen to reflect the three-in-one structure of the intelligence of nature found in Rik Ved. The first nucleotide initiates the codon sequence. It sets the direction for the intelligence represented in the codon and represents the Rishi value. The second nucleotide refines the direction set by the first codon, and links the first and third (representing the Devata value). The third nucleotide completes the codon, defines the knowledge precisely, and determines which amino acid will be used in the material structure of a protein (the third codon thus represents the Chhandas value). Together, the three represent a unique wholeness, greater than the sum of its parts and representing the Samhita value of the codon.

Furthermore, these 64 codons give rise to three levels of elaboration in the physiology:

1. Rishi—the coordinating and regulatory structures which embody continual knowingness within the body, including the brain and especially the limbic system.

2. Devata—the metabolic processes of transformation, by which the underlying intelligence within the DNA creates a physiology in its own image.

3. Chhandas—the solid structural components of the physiology.

At every stage of the process that gives rise to the body, moreover, the genetic code itself elaborates from a silent unity through three levels of expression:

Unity. The master code in the DNA itself, complete knowledge in a silent, integrated state (Samhita value).

1. The messenger RNA molecules, made from genetic code in the master DNA, which copy off and embody specific genes, particular packages of intelligence (Rishi value).

2. Molecules of transfer RNA, also made from the DNA's master code, which take hold of a particular amino acid and deliver it for attachment to the pattern of intelligence found on the messenger RNA (Devata value).

3. Formation of the final product, a physiological component, in the form of a protein molecule (Chhandas value).

The DNA contains all knowledge, silent, self-referral, and complete; the messenger RNA represents this silent intelligence in action; the transfer RNA is· the link between this intelligence and the raw materials available (amino acids); and the resulting protein molecules are the structural components used in building the body. In three sequential steps, the DNA's genetic code reaches out to make the body, without itself becoming embodied in any of the structural components that it creates.

From many standpoints, the 64 codons within the DNA are expressed at the three levels of Rishi, Devata, and Chhandas. Once again, 64 codons multiplied by three levels of expression give 192 fundamental elements out of which the entire human body is created. The structure of Rik Ved is paralleled in the structure of DNA. In the understandings of Maharishi Ayur-Ved, the Constitution of the Universe is lively within every cell in the body.

CONTACTING THE UNIFIED FIELD

The Constitution of the Universe may seem an abstract idea. Maharishi maintains, however, that every human being can personally experience this most basic level of nature. Every human being can verify, in fact, that the Constitution of the Universe—the unified field of natural law—is identical with the unified field of consciousness. The intelligence in the human mind is no different from the intelligence in nature; thus, the unified field of nature's intelligence can be directly experienced by any human being as the most unified level of his or her *own* intelligence. From this perspective, the most important capability of the human mind is that it can contact the unified field of natural law. To achieve this, a technology of conscious investigation must be used. In Maharishi's explanation, this is the most fundamental understanding of his Transcendental Meditation technique—it allows the human mind to settle down and identify itself with the silent basis of nature's functioning—the unified field of natural law.

The study of physics through objective investigation may not change the life of the physicist. But using the Transcendental Meditation technique to subjectively investigate the unified field *does* bring welcome change. Chapter Six detailed the research showing that Transcendental Meditation improves physical health, mental abilities, and psychological maturity. Maharishi explains that, by directly experiencing the unified field, one "imbibes" its infinite energy and intelligence. The mind and body come into accord with all the laws of nature at their source. Maharishi states,

> The functioning of transcendental pure consciousness is the functioning of natural law in its most settled state. The conscious human mind, identifying itself with this level of nature's functioning, gains the ability to perform in the style with which nature performs its activity at its most fundamental level.[16]

LIFE IN ACCORD WITH NATURAL LAW

If the body were to come fully into accord with the basic laws of nature that govern its functioning, then it should not fall sick. It should not degenerate. By the same token, if the mind were to come fully into accord with the basic laws of nature governing the intelligence in nature, then it should not make mistakes. It should achieve its desires more effortlessly. Research shows that evolution toward such ideal functioning does indeed occur with the regular practice of the Transcendental Meditation technique.

Maharishi emphasizes that this growth is *spontaneous.* The benefits of Transcendental Meditation are not the result of (1) thinking about the laws of nature, then (2) taking deliberate action. Instead, they result naturally, with no thought or effort, when the mind is in tune with natural law.

Even if you don't know how the electrons moving through a thin piece of wire can produce the light in a light bulb, you can still flick on the switch and enjoy the light. Even if it is impossible to have intellectual knowledge of all the infinite laws of nature, it is still possible to enjoy the practical benefits. As Maharishi summarizes,

> . . . the very methodology of gaining knowledge through Vedic Science is such that as one sees the knowledge of natural law on the intellectual level one begins to live that natural law in daily life in a most spontaneous way.[17]

LIFE IN ENLIGHTENMENT

For thousands of years, masters of the Vedic tradition have spoken of *enlightenment*. The term has often caused confusion, but we now have enough information to understand what enlightenment means. It does not mean possession of facts and figures—of intellectual knowledge. It means the light is on within. It means the individual mind is fully illumined by the infinite field of pure consciousness at the basis of nature.

Like a tree reaching its roots down to an underground reservoir, the human mind can settle down to experience this infinite field of pure intelligence. Maharishi explains that, by repeating this experience twice daily with Transcendental Meditation and the advanced TM-Sidhi program (see discussion in next chapter), the mind gains familiarity with this field. It gains the ability to maintain contact with the unified field of natural law even while going about its daily business:

> It's only in the beginning days of meditation that one has to meditate in order to experience that silent, quiet level of the mind, that state of pure consciousness. As we continue to alternate the experience of meditation with daily activity, the value of that pure consciousness is infused into the mind. The pure level of consciousness becomes stabilized in our awareness. And when that pure level . . . is a living reality even during daily activity, this is the state of enlightenment. This is life free from suffering, life when every thought and action is spontaneously correct.[18]

To make this point, Maharishi has used the analogy of dyeing a cloth. If a cloth is alternately dipped into yellow dye, then dried in the sun, it eventually becomes colorfast. If the mind is repeatedly dipped into pure consciousness, then brought out into the action of daily life, both mind and body eventually become fully habituated to that unbounded field of nature's intelligence. Contact with the unified field is maintained even during daily activity. The result is that life is lived 24 hours a day in perfect attunement with the laws of nature. As Maharishi has stated,

Transcendental Meditation and the TM-Sidhi program train the human brain physiology and human awareness to function completely in accord with the total potential of natural law and spontaneously exhibit natural law in daily life.[19]

One of Maharishi's favorite statements from the Vedic literature is, *Yatinam Brahm bhavati sarathih* ("For those whose minds are established in self-referral consciousness, the infinite organizing power of natural law becomes the charioteer"). In this state of life, daily living is said to be guided spontaneously by the laws of nature. When the mind is in tune with pure consciousness—the unified field of natural law—then thought and action are computed and conducted by all the laws of nature. When a great athlete goes "into the zone" for a few moments, every action is automatic and spontaneously right. This is a taste of enlightenment—life lived spontaneously in full accord with the laws of nature.

This state of enlightenment—when the individual mind is completely attuned to the infinite intelligence at the basis of nature—depends on subtle functioning of the body. In the human being, the mind depends on the brain. The quality of awareness depends on the quality of the physical machinery. This is why the quest for perfect health is integral to the quest for higher states of consciousness. The body and the nervous system must work perfectly for the mind to experience its full potential. Though consciousness is the basis of the physiology, ayurvedic vaidyas have always maintained that the body must be purified and perfectly tuned for that consciousness to shine through in its full glory. And this is why, with Maharishi Ayur-Ved, the same programs that produce better health also produce progress toward the highest states of consciousness. With this integrated system of natural health care, good health is grounded in growth toward enlightenment.

The result, Maharishi explains, is life in fulfillment. In his words, "This is how to live fullness in life—mistake-free life, disease-free life, problem-free life—life and daily living in full accord with Natural Law."[20]

FROM ENLIGHTENMENT TO PERFECT HEALTH

We have seen Maharishi's descriptions of the self-interacting dynamics of pure consciousness, and the way that these subtle fluctuations of intelligence give rise to the whole manifest creation. But we still need to know exactly how this understanding relates to the field of physical health. More to the point of this book, we need to know how it relates to the problem of free radicals.

It's obvious that the basic assumptions of Maharishi Ayur-Ved are quite different from those of modern medicine. Medical science thinks of the body as a complex machine: It is made of solid matter; it can get out of tune; it can be attacked by outside agents. To fix it when it is "broken," you shoot magic bullets (drugs), or cut and paste it together as if it were an auto engine in need of better wiring or a new piston.

Throughout most of this book, such a mechanical picture of the body would have sufficed. Molecules could be viewed as small agglomerations of solid matter, like BB's held together by magnetic attraction. The descriptions given by Maharishi, however, aided by the understandings from quantum mechanics, paint quite a different picture. The body is not a machine. It is an immensely complex flux of vibrations in an underlying, non-material field of pure intelligence. A molecule is not a collection of BB's, but a pattern of fluctuations created by the self-referral dynamism lively within pure intelligence.

If you drive a pole into the bed of a stream, standing it up straight, the water washing by will create a standing wave on the downstream side of the pole. Water that has separated to move around the pole rushes together again, creating a crest. This standing wave appears to have a constant shape and a continuous existence, but in fact, the water flowing through is new every instant.

Molecules can be thought of as standing waves. They appear solid and unchanging, but in fact, they are simply fluctuations of the underlying unified field. The individual atoms and particles come and go, replacing one another continually; only the underlying pattern remains the same.

The same is true for the body as a whole. Ninety-eight percent of the atoms in the body change every year. The atoms in bones, which are apparently so solid and permanent, are completely exchanged every three months. The body's skin is new every month, the stomach lining every four days, the surface cells that contact the food every five minutes.[21] In this flux of constant change, all that remains the same is the immensely complex standing wave in the underlying field of nature's intelligence. Consciousness is primary. The body is a pattern in the field of intelligence.

This means, among other things, that health care must change drastically. Superficial approaches will still have utility; if you break your leg, you'll still need a cast. But a truly effective health care system would not function only at this gross material level. Instead, it would also function at the most basic level of the laws of nature. It would function from both the surface and the depths.

The aim of Maharishi Ayur-Ved is to supply such an integrated approach. The next chapter details the many practical treatments available through Maharishi Ayur-Ved—twenty separate approaches for both body and mind. But in preparation, this chapter will conclude with an overview of Maharishi's theoretical understanding of the field of health. Effective practice must be based on sound theory.

THE MISTAKE OF THE INTELLECT

Maharishi begins his discussion of ayurveda with a definition of terms. The Sanskrit word *ayu* means life. *Ved* (VADE) or *Veda* (VADE-uh) means knowledge. Thus, ayurveda means the knowledge of life, or the science of life. [The final "a" in Sanskrit words is frequently dropped in pronunciation; over the years, Maharishi has sometimes reflected this in English transliterations and sometimes not; the quotations in this book have not been standardized, but appear as they were originally published. Some of Maharishi's books have been published in England, with such spellings as "fulfilment" and "ageing," which are also unchanged.]

In Maharishi Ayur-Ved, the analysis does not begin symptom by symptom, disease by disease. Instead, it focuses on the body's most fundamental level—the self-interacting dynamics of pure intelligence. In Maharishi's understanding, the etiology of all disease, and the basis of all cure, stems from this common source.

His logic begins by clarifying a key aspect of the interaction among Rishi, Devata, and Chhandas: He calls these three "intellectually conceived components" of the unified field of consciousness.[22]

By saying that the observer, the process of observation, and the observed are "intellectually conceived components," Maharishi is emphasizing that they are products of intellectual discrimination, rather than phenomena with absolute existence. Maharishi uses "intellect" to mean that faculty within the mind that draws distinctions. The intellect discriminates a knower, process of knowing, and known, when the reality is undifferentiated pure consciousness.

In Maharishi's explanation, there is no difficulty as long as the intellect does not get lost in its own discriminations. But as a sandstorm can hide the landscape, the swirl of dynamic interactions among Rishi, Devata, and Chhandas can hide the ultimate reality. The intellect gets lost in the complex, ever-changing vision of the world. Consciousness becomes *object-referral* instead of self-referral, lost in the masking value of Chhandas (the object of knowing). The glamour of the material creation fills the mind. The memory of the silent unity of consciousness—the Samhita of Rishi, Devata, and Chhandas—disappears. For this one-sided awareness, Maharishi uses the Sanskrit term *Pragya-aparadh*—the "mistake of the intellect."

Thus, the world we see—when devoid of simultaneous awareness of its basis in pure consciousness—is a grand illusion. Many physicists have come to the same conclusion. Realizing that the apparently solid objects around us are nothing but fluctuations in the non-material unified field, they have understood that material creation is an illusion created by our senses and our interpretations. This has been discussed at length by Sir James Jeans, Sir Arthur Eddington, Werner Heisenberg, Erwin Schroedinger, and many other prominent twentieth-century physicists. None, however, has stated the conclusion with greater vehemence than Paul Davies: "the . . . commonsense world of experience is a sham."[23]

RECONNECTING THE SURFACE WITH THE DEPTHS

In Maharishi Ayur-Ved, the solution is not to ignore this "sham," not to overlook the apparently solid physical body. The solution is to reconnect the surface with the depths. The goal, Maharishi states, ". . . is to keep the manifest states of creation in tune with the unmanifest state of pure knowledge."[24] This means that the essence of Maharishi Ayur-Ved is the "restoration of memory." The intellect, lost in its own discriminations, must remember its source once again—the undifferentiated unity of pure consciousness.

A gardener lost in the delight of eating his fruit must not forget to water the root of his tree. Only by remembering the most fundamental level of the tree can the gardener ensure the pleasures that come from the fruits. In the same way, Maharishi emphasizes that the manifest levels of life are rooted in the unmanifest, transcendental field of pure consciousness. As he states,

> . . . the unmanifest state and the manifesting process both have to remain in one's awareness. This is healthy awareness, enlightened consciousness of the individual, in which one does not forget the total potential of natural law when one is expressing oneself in limitations and boundaries.[25]

This is why meditation must be the basis for recovering health. The mind must leave behind the world of sense impressions and ceaseless activity. It must settle down deep within and experience its own silent source, Samhita, the unified field of pure consciousness—which is the most basic level of natural law. The Sanskrit word for memory is Smriti, and Maharishi has remarked,

> When the Smriti is lost, that is, when the memory of the unbounded is no more, then the [technology] of pure knowledge is introduced. This is the medicinal value of Ayur Veda which brings the functioning of the physiology back into accordance with the laws of nature and re-establishes that awareness which will continue to remember the totality of natural law.[26]

In this process of "remembering," meditation is the most important but not the only approach. All the numerous strategies of Maharishi Ayur-Ved have as their goal the reconnection of the material body with its basis in consciousness. Through every approach, the body is reminded of its source in consciousness. As Maharishi states, the secret of Maharishi Ayur-Ved is ". . . the secret of highly intensified mind-body coordination. And the secret of this mind-body coordination is the coordination of consciousness with itself."[27]

RESTORATION OF BALANCE

Put in other words, body must be balanced with mind. The objective must be balanced with the subjective. The outer must be balanced with the inner. In this sense, the importance of balance is strongly emphasized in every approach of Maharishi Ayur-Ved.

This fits well with the research evidence on free radicals. There is no need to, and no hope for, putting an end to free radicals. What the body must do is operate in a balanced way; free radicals must be balanced precisely by the defense and repair systems. In this situation, the destructive force of the free radicals can be offset by the creative force embodied in the repair mechanisms. Like a standing wave, the body can change constantly, yet remain intact and healthy.

This requirement for internal balance appears in many ways in all forms of life. The technical term is homeostasis. The human body, for example, uses elaborate strategies to dissipate excess heat, or to generate required heat—working always to keep the balance near 98.6° Fahrenheit, the optimum temperature for the biochemical reactions necessary for human life. Similarly, for those same reactions to occur, the body must maintain the proper pH level—the proper balance between acidity and alkalinity.

Such balance is indispensable to life. Given the importance of homeostasis in the body, it comes as no surprise that in Maharishi Ayur-Ved a perfectly healthy body is viewed as one in perfect balance. But the conception of balance in Maharishi Ayur-Ved is rooted much more deeply than in modern medicine.

Awareness lost in the apparently physical world is considered to be the most fundamental imbalance—and this imbalance is considered the source of all discomfort and "dis-ease." "Balance is a state of satisfaction," Maharishi indicates. "Deviation from balance is dissatisfaction. Pain and suffering result from imbalances."[28]

An imbalance in acidity means the body's cells cannot take in nutrients properly. An imbalance of free radicals creates havoc in the physiology. Yet, in the course of solely outer-directed living, Maharishi indicates, the upsurge of such imbalance is inevitable. The unified field embodies perfect balance; its various components exhibit what physicists term supersymmetry. But the very process by which the unified field gives rise to the world is a process physicists call spontaneous symmetry breaking. Perfect balance gives rise to imbalance spontaneously. The same process is seen in the mechanics of consciousness, as Maharishi remarks:

> We have seen how the three-fold structure of the Veda—Rishi, Devata, and Chhandas—breaks from their unity. This is the fundamental feat of spontaneous dynamical symmetry breaking, as it is called in quantum field theory. Because this breaking of symmetry is a natural phenomenon, imbalance is also a natural phenomenon. . . . Anywhere in the process of manifestation of intelligence into matter or in the reaction of matter with matter, anywhere in those space-time boundaries that the self-referral condition is unavailable, there is pain and suffering.[29]

Maharishi asserts that spontaneous imbalance can be rectified. The imbalances in the manifest physiology can be corrected by reconnecting to the perfect balance of the unified field. As he states,

> The unified field is perfectly balanced because its status is self-referral, its activity is self-interacting. It cannot be probed by anything from outside. It cannot be disturbed. It is a state of eternal balance, which is the ideal of balance. . . . It keeps natural activity completely balanced and operating with such great precision that there is absolute precision in nature's functioning.[30]

When the memory of pure consciousness is restored, then within the physiological *expressions* of pure consciousness, balance is also restored. The perfect symmetry of the silent, nonmaterial unified field is infused into the activity of the apparently material body. Maharishi explains that, "The knowledge contained in Ayurveda of restoring balance to an imbalanced state is from that absolute state of knowledge about how self-referral consciousness assumes material form."[31]

AGING AND IMMORTALITY

In Maharishi's understanding, the ultimate result produced by such a profoundly balanced approach to health care can be far beyond anything dreamed of in modern medical science. If perfect balance can be maintained in cellular functioning, if perfect balance can be maintained between free radicals and the defenses against them, then it is not obvious, even in the Western tradition of medicine, why the body should age and deteriorate.

As ever, Maharishi bases his understanding on the mechanics within the unified field of intelligence. The unity of pure consciousness, Samhita, is a constant reality. Likewise, the interplay of Rishi, Devata, and Chhandas continually occurs. Both are inherent in the nature of consciousness: It *is* a unified whole, yet it must ever know itself. There was never a time before the unity diversified into knower, process of knowing, and known. There will never be a time when the 3-in-1 mechanics will cease to take place. In the Vedic literature, the manifest universe is said to be "beginningless" and "without end."

In terms of physical health, Maharishi has explained,

> Rishi, Devata, and Chhandas in their coordinated value maintain Samhita . . . in an immortal state. . . . Pure knowledge is immortal. The organizing power of nature inherent in the structure of pure knowledge is immortal. Thus balance is immortal, and if, through the knowledge of Ayurveda, one maintains balance in the physiology, mind, and behavior, then that is the direction of long life....[32]

There is certainly no way to maintain health indefinitely by diagnosing and curing disease after disease. Life can't be maintained on the basis of constant vigilance for symptoms. In Maharishi Ayur-Ved, the life span is said to depend on the level of refinement attained by both mind and body. In Maharishi's understanding, the body will age with every mistake, with every violation of natural law. The only way to avoid mistakes is to align oneself with all the laws of nature at their source—and gain the support of natural law for every thought and action. As Maharishi explains,

> Spontaneity of action in accordance with all the laws of nature is the only way to eliminate the process of ageing. If there is violation of even a few laws of nature, then ageing will continue breathing in life. The total value of natural law has to become a living reality, no aspect of natural law must be violated—then immortality will be a continuum.[33]

INTELLIGENCE AND MOLECULES

In the first two parts of this book, we saw that free radicals pose a profound challenge to health and longevity. Only a comprehensive and deeply-rooted health care approach could possibly counter such an integral threat.

We now have good reason to believe that Maharishi Ayur-Ved provides such a comprehensive and deeply-rooted approach. Maharishi Ayur-Ved goes beyond the molecular level where free radicals operate and bases its theories and techniques on the underlying field of pure intelligence. From the perspective of both modern science and Maharishi's Vedic Science, this appears to be the most fundamental possible standpoint for creating better health.

Without consideration of this underlying field of intelligence, in fact, the dance of molecules in every cell seems inexplicable. Billions of molecules jiggle and bang through countless lightning-fast reactions—and somehow an entire walled "city" emerges, with energy plants, waste treatment facilities, manufacturing centers, and rapid communications. The wholeness of the cell is so spectacularly intelligent. How can it possibly result from the random jostlings of mindless, material molecules?

It all makes sense if we adjust our eyes to see the underlying pattern rather than the place holders. The swirls and eddies near the edges of a stream can be seen in the motions of leaves floating on the surface. The swirls and eddies in the underlying field of consciousness can be seen in the movements of molecules as they interact in the cell. To change the metaphor, a child can slide a magnet under the top of the dinner table and pull the silverware around. The stronger the magnet, the more easily the silverware moves. Similarly, if the underlying field of intelligence is lively, then the molecules in every cell should be swirled smoothly through their actions and reactions.

In Maharishi's explanation, the infinitely dynamic interplay of Rishi, Devata, and Chhandas produces a whirlpool in the unified field of nature's intelligence. This whirlpool gives rise to an infinite variety of waves, underlying the infinite variety of the manifest creation. In his view, every molecule is a fluctuation of this underlying intelligence.

THE LAW OF LEAST ACTION

But why does this approach produce such unprecedented control of free radicals? One answer involves a principle fundamental to the intelligence of natural law—the *law of least action*. Nature always does everything with the least possible effort—a principle that has been called the "cosmic law of laziness." Water always flows downhill. Chemical reactions always take place with the least possible expenditure of energy. Nature operates by the path of least resistance.

When the mind and body come more fully into alignment with the unified field of natural law, they should therefore come more fully into accord with the law of least action. This should mean that the psychophysiology operates more easily, with less effort and strain. We have seen research that indicates this is true. People who practice Transcendental Meditation are less anxious and more relaxed. Their physiologies do not strain as much and so (largely because their electron transport chains are not overworked) they produce fewer free radicals. Health improves dramatically.

We have understood this as physiological stress reduction. But it can also be understood as life more completely in accord with natural law.

In addition, Maharishi Amrit Kalash scavenges free radicals that do get created—and it does so in a manner that is completely natural. It takes advantage of nature's own synergistic anti-oxidant systems created in the plant kingdom. These systems are infused with the same intelligence that underlies the human body and everything else in creation. Moreover, the precise plants used in these herbal formulations have been chosen and combined by human intelligences which are themselves said to be enlightened—in tune with the pure field of intelligence at the basis of nature. Though it is possible to argue that artificial or isolated ingredients selected through the trial-and-error method of objective science could fight free radicals as well as Maharishi Amrit Kalash, the research evidence to date indicates otherwise. Nature's law of least action has apparently been upheld in this case also; MAK scavenges free radicals as well as a much-researched anti-oxidant drug and the best-known free radical-quenching vitamins—in amounts one thousand times as small.

The research we have seen in Part Two indicates that these natural approaches to free radical management produce dramatic improvements in health—and reductions in health care costs. Now these practical findings can be theoretically understood. In the perspective of Maharishi Ayur-Ved, to rebalance the body and minimize the threat from free radicals, we must restore our connection with nature's intelligence. We must live in accord with natural law.

Notes

1. Sharma PV, ed., *Charak Samhita, Vol II*, Chikitsasthanam 1.4.57 (Chaukhambha Orientalia, Varanasi, India, 1983), p. 34

2. Maharishi Mahesh Yogi, *Maharishi's Vedic Science*, Lesson One (Pre-publication manuscript), p. 12

3. Maharishi Mahesh Yogi, *Life Supported by Natural Law* (Age of Enlightenment Press, Washington, DC, 1986), p. 34

4. Ibid

5. Ibid, p. 28

6. Ibid, p. 109

7. Ibid, p. 25-6

8. Ibid, p. 75

9. Ibid, p. 33

10. Ibid

11. Ibid, p. 30

12. Hagelin JS, *Mod Sci Ved Sci* 1(1)(1987): 58

13. Ibid, p. 77

14. Ibid, p. 60

15. Ibid, p. 59

16. Maharishi, *Life* (see note 3), pp. 31

17. Ibid, p. 34-5

18. Oates RM Jr., *Celebrating the Dawn* (G. P. Putnam's Sons, New York, 1976), pp. 33-4

19. Maharishi, *Life* (see note 3), p. 32

20. Maharishi, *Maharishi's* (see note 2), p. 9

21. Dossey L, *Space, Time & Medicine* (Shambhala, Boston and London, 1985), p. 74

22. Maharishi, *Life* (see note 3), pp. 25-6

23. Davies P, *Superforce: The Search for a Grand Unified Theory of Nature* (Touchstone, Simon & Schuster, New York, 1985), p. 37

24. *Proceedings Int'l Conf Sci Cons Ageing* (Seelisberg, Switzerland, 1980), p. 17

25. Ibid

26. Ibid, p. 16

27. Maharishi, *Life* (see note 3), p. 25

28. Ibid, p. 110

29. Ibid, pp. 110-1
30. Ibid, p. 109
31. Ibid, p. 47
32. Ibid, p. 114
33. *Proceedings* (see note 24), p. 19

CHAPTER NINE

The Twenty Approaches of Maharishi Ayur-Ved

If you walk into most medical offices and receive a cancer diagnosis, you will almost surely be assigned some type of attack therapy. The current medical model looks at the body and disease process from a materialistic point of view. This model views cancer cells as foreign objects. The goal of the therapy is to attack these foreign objects and annihilate them. The treatments are combative—surgery, radiation, chemotherapy—as if disease can best be treated by carpet bombing.

Unfortunately, such destructive treatments are rarely so tightly targeted as to spare healthy tissues. The result is destruction of normal structure and function—what we know as side effects. Because of the power of these medical weapons, the side effects are often severe, and may even be life-threatening. For example, radiation and chemotherapy commonly weaken the immune system, making the patient susceptible to infections and other diseases—even new cancers.

Maharishi Ayur-Ved takes a completely different approach. Rather than focusing on foreign objects and destructive weaponry, it focuses on the non-material field of intelligence which underlies and orchestrates the functioning of the body.

Faced with cancer, Maharishi Ayur-Ved does not aim solely to get rid of the tumor. It also aims to reinstate the normal flow of intelligence—from the underlying field through the DNA and on to every process in the cell. This approach is said to enliven the body's vitality, immune system, and self-repair mechanisms. Maharishi Ayur-Ved takes the consciousness paradigm and translates it into practical action.

Medical doctors trained in Maharishi Ayur-Ved point out that it is complementary to allopathic medicine. Especially in chronic ailments, conventional medical therapies can be employed in conjunction with Maharishi Ayur-Ved. Experience has shown that such treatment is often more effective, with fewer side effects. But the most important role of ayurvedic medicine, traditionally, has been prevention. Don't let people fall sick in the first place. Don't put them in a position where destructive therapies must be considered at all.

TWENTY WAYS TO CONTROL FREE RADICALS

From the free radical perspective, the goal is to control them and all their damage—from cancer to heart disease and aging. To do so requires a fundamental restructuring of the body's functioning. Free radical creation is integral to the biochemical operation of every cell. Only a systematic refinement in the way the body works can hope to produce a major effect on the free radical problem.

This helps explain why Maharishi Ayur-Ved employs a wide range of subtle technologies. The intent is to fine-tune both body and mind. The formula is to positively affect psychophysiological metabolism in as many ways as possible.

As we have seen, every experience we have affects our health. We are re-made every instant by the food we eat, the air we breathe, the work we do, the conversations we have, the thoughts we entertain, the emotions we go through. If you have a hard day at the office, you can feel the tension-producing effects of catecholamines. If you see a magnificent sunset, you can feel the settling and satisfying effects of serotonin and other neuropeptides. The limbic system metabolizes every experience we have, recreating our body as we go.

The twenty approaches of Maharishi Ayur-Ved take advantage of this rich interaction between experience and physiology. Doctors need not be confined to the use of pills and needles, surgical knives and radiation machines. The bodies of their patients can be changed, subtly but powerfully, by sights and sounds, by thoughts and feelings, by action and by silence. By taking a richly comprehensive approach that addresses the psychophysiology in many different ways, the underlying patterns of intelligence can be rebalanced and refined.

In Maharishi's understanding, at that level where the unified field of natural law assumes physiological form, the restoration of perfect balance allows the effortless and accurate transformation of intelligence into matter. For this reason, the psychophysiology must once again be brought into accord with the most basic field of intelligence in nature. Instead of attacking the body, in other words, Maharishi Ayur-Ved aims to remind it of its own source.

MAHARISHI AYUR-VED

This "new" system, of course, is not new at all. Ayurveda is the world's oldest and most comprehensive system of natural health care. It is widely used in India, and recognized by the World Health Organization as an effective traditional health care system.

In recent years, Maharishi has worked to revive this ancient knowledge in its completeness. He has continually consulted with leading ayurvedic vaidyas, including Dr. B.D. Triguna, past president of the All-India Ayurveda Congress, and Director of the National Academy for Ayurveda. It was during conversations with Dr. Triguna that Maharishi first made the decision to begin his revival of the ancient ayurvedic health care system. The goal Maharishi and Dr. Triguna set at that time: the creation of a disease-free society.

The result of this collaborative effort is Maharishi Ayur-Ved, which, despite its ancient roots, is notably modern in its systematic and scientific approach. The significant contribution of Maharishi Ayur-Ved is that it treats disease at its source, rather than merely pacifying symptoms. It focuses on prevention, though it also provides treatment. It is health care—care that promotes health.

Maharishi Ayur-Ved works by correcting subtle imbalances in the body before they erupt as disease. By correcting these imbalances, it strengthens the body's immune system and innate homeostatic self-repair mechanisms, so the body naturally resists disease. Many medical doctors have now taken training in Maharishi Ayur-Ved. They comment that the treatments are not only efficacious, but also easy to apply, free from side effects, and notably cost effective.

In this chapter we will introduce the basic diagnostic concept of Maharishi Ayur-Ved, and briefly review the twenty approaches for "treatment"—or, more precisely, for creating balance in the physiology. These pages are intended only as an overview, to give some appreciation of the main ideas and some indication of the way in which the system promises a comprehensive approach to the problem of free radicals. For details, consult a physician trained in Maharishi Ayur-Ved (see phone numbers listed in *Resources*, page 330).

THE CONCEPT OF BODY TYPE

Doctors trained in Maharishi Ayur-Ved do not focus on superficial aches and pains. Rather they monitor and address the most fundamental levels of the psychophysiology. At the most basic level are the three components of the unified field of intelligence: Rishi (knower), Devata (process of knowing), and Chhandas (known). Maharishi Ayur-Ved indicates that when the self-referral interactions of Rishi, Devata, and Chhandas have become sufficiently dynamic and complex, the three appear as *doshas*—subtle metabolic principles that underlie every activity of the human physiology. These three doshas are Vat (VAHT), Pitt, and Kaph (KAHF). To best understand how the twenty approaches of Maharishi Ayur-Ved achieve their purposes, it will be beneficial to understand these three basic doshas.

Psychophysiological body types: In the teachings of Maharishi Ayur-Ved, everyone is born with a particular mixture of Vat, Pitt, and Kaph, and in each person the exact proportions vary. Thus, from the doctor's viewpoint, patients are not all the same. Each has a different constitution—known as the psychophysiological body type. Each body type has a propensity toward certain diseases, and an affinity for certain cures. To give accurate diagnoses and effective cures, a doctor must first know the patient's basic constitution, or body type—the relative proportions of the underlying doshas.

In Western medicine, constitutional typing has received occasional attention. The concept of typologically discrete differences in human psychophysiology was introduced to Western medicine by Sheldon in the last century. More recently, Friedman and Rosenman developed the concept of the Type A coronary-prone behavior pattern. Research has shown that behavioral differences between Type A and Type B individuals are matched by physiological differences in cortisol, growth hormone, testosterone, and catecholamines. Some interest has been shown in these ideas, but the concepts are clearly provisional. Recent research has revealed, for example, that the only aspect of Type A behavior that actually correlates with heart disease is anger and hostility—whether expressed or repressed.[1]

The ayurvedic approach to body typing, on the other hand, has been utilized for thousands of years. It is detailed and sophisticated, involving ten different combinations of Vat, Pitt, and Kaph. The body type is determined through a detailed history and physical examination, including pulse diagnosis as a central feature.

The three doshas: The most obvious principles of ayurvedic body typing can be easily grasped. If you go to get a new driver's license and watch people trapped in a long line, you can get some idea of their underlying dosha make-up. People who appear anxious and worried, who fidget, look over their shoulders, look at their watches, wring their hands—are likely to be predominantly Vat. People who look red-faced and angry, who glare piercingly around, push for position, yell at the clerks—are likely to be predominantly Pitt. People who seem content and at ease, who may look a bit plump or stolid, who wait patiently, who may look to sit down—are likely to be predominantly Kaph.

The three doshas have distinctive characteristics, and impart a particular style or tone to everyone's psychophysiology. Vaidyas maintain, for example, that an excess of Pitt leads to anger and hostility. It is thus interesting to note that research using the Jenkins Activity Survey shows that people with a strong Pitt body type tend to be Type A personalities. On the other hand, people with a Kaph body type (associated by vaidyas with physical and mental steadiness) tend to be Type B personalities. The ayurvedic classifications thus help to explain modern discoveries about psychophysiological type.[2]

According to Maharishi Ayur-Ved, the doshas are the most basic controllers of the psychophysiology. When they are in balance—that is, when each is in the correct proportion for that particular individual—then health is optimal. Vat dosha governs movement, such as breathing and blood circulation. Pitt governs heat, metabolism, energy production, and other chemical reactions. Kaph governs physical substance and fluid balance, the structural basis of the body. All must work smoothly together to produce optimal health.

Balance in the doshas: The primary goal of Maharishi Ayur-Ved, therefore, is to restore and maintain the proper balance of all three doshas for each person. Such doshic balance enhances homeostatic balance in the body's biochemistry and favors self-repair mechanisms over free radical damage. If a person's underlying body type is, for example, 60% Vat, 30% Pitt and 10% Kaph, then these proportions should be maintained. Each dosha should maintain its optimum level; it should not become too weak or too strong (aggravated). When doshas become aggravated or excessive, this especially creates imbalance, and that imbalance can lead to disease. Whichever dosha dominates in the original body type is the dosha most likely to become aggravated and out of balance.

The qualities of Vat: Each dosha, in proper balance, generates admirable qualities in both body and mind. By nature, the Vat psychological traits are imagination, sensitivity, spontaneity, and resiliency. Other signs of balanced Vat include:

- Mental alertness
- Proper formation of body tissues
- Normal elimination
- Sound sleep
- Sense of exhilaration

Vat can be aggravated fairly easily, however. Many things aggravate Vat, including stress, mental or physical fatigue and lack of sleep, traveling, alcohol and smoking, food that is cold, raw, or dry, extreme dieting or skipping meals, and cold, dry, windy weather. Once Vat has gone out of balance, it can give rise to a wide variety of symptoms:

- Anxiety, worry
- Insomnia, restlessness
- Low appetite
- Dry or rough skin

- Constipation
- Low energy
- Tension headaches
- Intolerance of cold
- Aching joints
- Muscle spasms, low back pain
- Underweight

The qualities of Pitt: By nature, the balanced Pitt type is intellectual, confident, enterprising, and joyous. Other signs of balanced Pitt include:

- Normal heat and thirst mechanisms
- Strong digestion
- Lustrous complexion
- Effective speaking
- Contentment

Pitt can be driven out of balance as well. Pitt is the dosha of heat, and it can be aggravated by stress that causes anger, frustration, or resentment, by constant pressure and time deadlines, by food that is spicy, oily, salty, or sour, by food or water that is impure, by weather that is hot and humid, and by excessive sun. Once Pitt has gone out of balance, it can give rise to:

- Hostility, irritability, resentment
- Self-criticism
- Rashes, skin inflammation
- Peptic ulcer, heartburn
- Excessive body heat, intolerance of heat
- Visual problems
- Premature graying or baldness

The qualities of Kaph: By nature, the balanced Kaph type is calm, sympathetic, courageous, forgiving, and loving. Other Kaph traits include:

- Muscular strength
- Vitality and stamina
- Strong immunity
- Affection, generosity, dignity
- Stability of mind
- Healthy, normal joints

Kaph can be aggravated by gaining a great deal of weight, by food that is heavy, fatty, and sweet (including dairy products like cheese, milk, and ice cream), by stress that causes feelings of insecurity or being unwanted, by relationships that cause dependency or overprotectiveness, by excess sleep, and by weather that is cold, damp, and snowy. Once Kaph is aggravated, it can give rise to:

- Dullness, sleepiness, and mental inertia
- Depression
- Attachment, greed, or possessiveness
- Intolerance of cold and damp
- Sinus congestion, chest congestion, frequent colds
- High cholesterol
- Weight gain, fluid retention
- Diabetes

(Keep in mind that the traits and symptoms listed here are general guidelines.)

Balancing doshas and controlling free radicals: Stated simply, the goal of Maharishi Ayur-Ved is to keep the doshas in balance. For people who are not seriously ill, it is relatively easy to keep a rough balance. Regular meditation, plus simple changes in diet and daily routine (adjusted as the seasons change), will usually do the trick. But the aim of Maharishi Ayur-Ved is not so inexact. It intends not just a rough balance in the doshas and reasonably good health, but perfect balance and ideal health—a "friction-free" style of functioning that can support extremely long life.

As we have seen, no imbalance in the body is more destructive than a free radical overhang. In the view of ayurvedic vaidyas, the way to keep free radicals in balance is to keep the doshas in balance. Dr. B.D. Triguna maintains, in fact, that dosha balance and free radical balance are two ways of talking about the same thing. Ayurvedic descriptions of the damage done by imbalanced doshas parallel modern descriptions of the damage done by excess free radicals. He quotes from an ancient ayurvedic text, the *Shushrut Samhita*, which says,

> When functioning normally, Vat, Pitt, and Kaph constitute the body, protect the body, and are called dhatus. When vitiated [out of balance] Vat, Pitt, and Kaph roam in the body, and wherever they find deficiency, they create disease, and are called doshas.[3]

A single underlying imbalance creates a myriad of diseases. It is not the cause that varies from disease to disease, but underlying weakness at various places in the physiology. The descriptions do have an intriguing similarity.

In any event, objective evidence has clearly shown that techniques of Maharishi Ayur-Ved, while aiming at rebalancing the doshas, control free radical damage far more effectively than any other approach that has been tested so far. For this dual purpose, it offers a wide range of techniques to fine-tune mind, body, and the relationship between the two. Following is a brief overview of the twenty different approaches to achieve this perfect balance and bring free radical damage under control.

CONSCIOUSNESS

The central goal of the revival of ayurveda as Maharishi Ayur-Ved is to return consciousness to its rightful role at the basis of healing and perfect health. The physicist Max Planck said, "I believe consciousness is primary. I believe matter is derivative from consciousness."[4] For thousands of years, this has been the central understanding in the classical texts on ayurveda. The body is generated by the self-interacting dynamics of consciousness. Attention to consciousness must be the doctor's first priority.

In recent centuries, however, this focus on consciousness had faded from ayurveda. According to Maharishi, the major reason for this was the incorrect practice of meditation. Gradually the idea took hold that meditation is difficult and requires intense concentration. This meant that meditation could only be practiced by a gifted and dedicated few, living in mountains and caves far from the distractions of daily life. Given this misunderstanding, doctors could not prescribe meditation. No one would practice it.

When Maharishi began his teaching in the mid-1950s, his main focus was to reverse this misunderstanding of meditation. He emphasized that meditation is actually effortless and natural—in tune with nature's law of least action. Anyone who can run, can walk, he said, and anyone who can walk, can stand still. If the mind is running rapidly, it can slow down naturally and eventually become silent. It is only necessary to give the mind the correct angle, then let go. In Maharishi's words,

> The Transcendental Meditation technique is easy because it is natural. Evolution is natural to life. It is the natural tendency of the mind to settle down to more refined levels. This is why we know that if a technique is hard, it is unnatural. If it is hard, it is against the natural tendency of life. For centuries past, the message has been broadcast that meditation is difficult, that it is for some chosen few in life. But the reason for that has just been lack of guidance, lack of proper guidance.[5]

Doctors can and do prescribe Transcendental Meditation. It has proven so easy to learn that even ten-year-old children can do it. In addition, as we have seen, its health benefits have been verified by hundreds of research studies. And because it requires no religious beliefs, and no changes in philosophy or lifestyle, it can be practiced by people from every culture and walk of life.

Turning attention within: This effortless practice is intended to refine human awareness. When we first step out in the sunlight, we may not see much until our eyes adjust. The Vedic tradition has supplied systematic meditation techniques to allow our inner eye to adjust to the inner light—to the fundamental levels of intelligence within the mind.

Ordinarily, the human mind moves only outward through the senses to contact the apparently physical world. The mind does not commonly go inward, toward its own source. This habit of outer attention does not cultivate refined levels of human awareness. Without the regular practice of meditation, Maharishi explains,

> . . . our senses may be capable only of the gross, outer experiences of daily life. And if we experience the gross levels for a long time the capacity for subtle experience is rusted because the machinery is not used. When the finer faculties of experience are not used, then life becomes dry and dull, brittle and tense.[6]

The practice of the Transcendental Meditation technique is intended to refine the awareness. Maharishi indicates that, during the practice of Transcendental Meditation, the mind dives beneath the conscious level of thoughts and perceptions. It begins to experience its own inner nature. When the mind experiences a thought in its early, less concrete states, it is experiencing the process that *creates* finished thoughts, instead of experiencing only the finished thoughts themselves. Ultimately, this process of refinement culminates when the mind transcends all thought activity. It then experiences pure consciousness—the silent source of all mental activity. In Maharishi's description,

When consciousness is flowing out into the field of thoughts and activity, it identifies itself with many things, and this is how experience takes place. Consciousness coming back onto itself [during Transcendental Meditation] gains an integrated state, because consciousness in itself is completely integrated. This is pure consciousness, or transcendental consciousness. From this basic level of life emerge all fields of existence, all kinds of intelligence.[7]

Transcendental Meditation allows the mind to settle down deep within itself. There it directly *experiences* the most basic level of pure consciousness. Maharishi emphasizes that this is not just thinking about the unified field. This is immersion *within* the unified field. As we saw in Chapter Six, this experience of pure consciousness produces many benefits for both body and mind. The experience of deep relaxation and pure consciousness feeds new stimuli into the limbic region of the brain. Everywhere in the body, cell receptors receive the molecular news of the fourth state of consciousness. The body's structure and activity are transformed.

The TM-Sidhi program: In his Vedic Science, Maharishi offers additional technologies of consciousness. The most widely used is the TM-Sidhi program, a series of advanced meditation techniques. If the Transcendental Meditation technique is like diving to the deepest level of pure intelligence, the TM-Sidhi program is like underwater swimming— moving around *within* the field of pure intelligence. Established deep within, the mind entertains particular impulses or formulas (the Sanskrit word is Sutras). Each Sutra gives a particular direction to pure consciousness. It stirs and enlivens that most basic level of natural law. Maharishi has described the process in this way:

The TM-Sidhi program trains the conscious mind to function in this field of pure consciousness. In the TM-Sidhi program one takes a Sutra and it dissolves, and then another Sutra and it dissolves. At that point when the first Sutra has dissolved but the second has not yet emerged is the experience of the self-referral state of consciousness. In this state the previous Sutra is transforming itself into the next. The gap between the two Sutras is a self-referral state of awareness, but it has that dynamism of one transforming into the other. . . . Physicists call this the self-interacting quality of the unified field. Those who practice the TM-Sidhi program experience that self-interacting quality as one value transforms into another value.[8]

When the mind is trapped in superficial awareness of the surface appearance of the world, it sees only objects and action. This limited experience is all that can be metabolized by the body. Transcendental Meditation and the TM-Sidhi program expand this experience. The mind experiences not only objects, but also the subject—the deepest level of its own nature. It knows not only action, but also silence—the unbounded consciousness at the basis of activity. The outward stroke of the mind, experiencing the world created by natural law, is balanced by an inward stroke, experiencing the *source* of natural law. Maharishi Ayur-Ved maintains that this dual experience balances the doshas, and thereby prevents disease before it can arise.

The research on Transcendental Meditation demonstrates that it reduces health care utilization in every category of disease. This evidence upholds Maharishi Ayur-Ved's consciousness-based approach to health. For the first time it is clear that a health care system based on consciousness provides a powerful tool for prevention.

RASAYANAS

Maharishi Amrit Kalash (MAK-4 and MAK-5) are *rasayanas*—a class of herbal food supplements designed to enhance general well-being. The classical texts on ayurveda say that rasayanas promote vitality, stamina, resistance to disease, and longevity. The research reported earlier showed that MAK-4 and MAK-5 are markedly more effective at fighting free radicals than other proven free radical scavengers. This quality on its own would make them an important addition to the diet. But Maharishi Amrit Kalash is said to have far greater effects on both mind and body than simply stopping free radicals—and the research has shown that they also help reverse cancer, prevent platelet aggregation, and stimulate the activity of the immune system.

Because MAK is so complex in its molecular makeup, the exact mechanisms are difficult to identify through objective research. But Maharishi indicates that the effects of MAK are not all on the objective, material level, in any event. In his understanding, MAK works from the field level of nature, that level where, as we have seen, solid matter has evaporated and only intelligence remains.

On the one hand, Maharishi Amrit Kalash is an herbal food supplement—an apparently obvious example of the stuff of the world. But as Sir Arthur Eddington said, the stuff of the world is mind-stuff. Every molecule in Maharishi Amrit Kalash is actually a particular pattern of intelligence.

If the body is suffering disease, then the intelligence in the body is out of balance somewhere. Maharishi maintains that such an imbalance can be corrected by inserting patterns of intelligence that originate outside the body. He explains,

> The body of everything is governed by natural law, including the bodies of animals, trees, and herbs. All the different structures in the relative field, including our bodies, have their own impulses of natural law. . . . If imbalance arises anywhere, then Ayurveda suggests exactly the impulses to correct the imbalance, in whatever herb, root, bark, fruit, or wherever they are found. The same impulses which make the . . . teeth, the skin, the bone—the same kind of impulses, wherever they are found in nature, are brought and applied. The restoration of balance, which means the curing of sicknesses, is brought about . . . . The laws of nature found in the herbs and those in the body are put together and balance is restored.[9]

If disease is ultimately at the level of underlying intelligence, then only treatment with patterns, or impulses, of intelligence will be most effective. Superficial treatments may have some effect. You can lower a patient's temperature with aspirin, decrease inflammation with steroids, lower blood pressure with anti-hypertensive drugs. But to fine-tune the deepest imbalances that occur as the unified field first undergoes symmetry breaking, only a profound understanding of the mechanics of natural law will suffice, and only a delicate and precise set of procedures will produce a natural and lasting cure. In Maharishi's words,

> Ayurveda achieves these purposes through knowledge of the impulses of intelligence or consciousness which have taken some material form. Through knowledge of the infinitely balancing impulses of intelligence available in some herb or root or fruit, Ayurveda provides a cure for any imbalance that has developed in the body. In Ayurveda these impulses of intelligence are incorporated to heal the ailment, and, by being incorporated in the conscious mind, bring about the repair of any damage which has dismantled mind-body coordination in any part of the body.[10]

Through rasayanas, then, the body is able to directly metabolize the patterns of intelligence needed to restore optimal functioning. Rasayanas need not wait for the limbic system to create new molecules. In the view of Maharishi Ayur-Ved, rasayanas provide those molecules directly, and reset physiological sequences that have gone awry.

This analysis underlies the broad-based claims for MAK's effectiveness. These claims have now been backed up by broad-based evidence of MAK's benefits. As with meditation, research evidence has now shown that rasayanas can make a major contribution to better health.

HERBAL FOOD SUPPLEMENTS

In addition to the rasayanas, which can help everyone, Maharishi Ayur-Ved uses specific herbal supplements to treat specific dosha imbalances. Knowledge in this area (as well as for rasayanas) includes which plants and parts of plants to use, when to collect them, how to store them, and how to prepare them. Preparation typically involves the fine grinding procedure described earlier, which enhances the digestibility of the mixture.

As the last chapter explained, each molecule in these herbs is actually an impulse of intelligence, a particular "standing wave" in the underlying field of consciousness. When carefully chosen, these match the impulses of intelligence in different parts of the human body. When the mind and body go out of balance, there are disruptions in the natural sequence that leads from pure intelligence to DNA, RNA, proteins, and on to the complete physiology. One such sequence produces liver cells, for example, another the heart. Anywhere a sequence is disrupted, disease can appear in that particular part of the body.

The herbal preparations of Maharishi Ayur-Ved are said to provide the correct impulse to "reset" a particular sequence, to build a continuous bridge again from the unified field of pure intelligence all the way to the manifest, surface-level expressions of the body. We have mentioned the research showing that Maharishi Amrit Kalash encourages cancer cells to restore themselves to the healthy, functioning cells they once were. Ayurvedic vaidyas indicate that this process of re-differentiation means that the correct sequence has again been restored. When the sequence is intact, the intelligence flows smoothly, the doshas are rebalanced, and health is restored.

PANCHAKARMA: PHYSIOLOGICAL PURIFICATION

Panchakarma is one of Maharishi Ayur-Ved's major approaches for both prevention and treatment of disease. On one level, panchakarma presents a new, soothing, and enlivening experience for the body to metabolize. Panchakarma includes sophisticated massages with medicated oil, heat treatments with herbalized steam, inhalation therapy to cleanse sinuses and lungs, and a variety of purgative and eliminative therapies. The experience is both relaxing and invigorating.

However, panchakarma has a more specific purpose: to eliminate physiological impurities from the system. Impurities, toxins, and cellular waste products can derange cell functioning and disrupt health. If left untreated, such impurities can lead to degenerative disorders and life-threatening disease. Panchakarma is designed to purify the body and thereby avert the development of disease. Its treatments are designed to first loosen impurities from bodily tissues, then eliminate them from the body altogether.

Each treatment is individualized depending on the patient's body type and which doshas are imbalanced. It is recommended that adults take these purification treatments once each season, to keep the physiological machinery functioning properly.

Research: Panchakarma has also been scientifically investigated here at The Ohio State University, in collaboration with Dr. Edwards Smith and other investigators at MIU in Fairfield, Iowa. As this book has shown, free radicals are among the most toxic impurities the body must face. Although the tiny oxy radicals do not persist long enough for their levels to be tested, lipid peroxides (the damaged fatty molecules that can deteriorate into more free radicals) do have a measurable life span. In fact, as we have seen, measurement of lipid peroxide levels in the blood is often used as a measure of overall free radical activity in the body.

In theory, panchakarma should reduce lipid peroxide levels. One aspect of panchakarma involves increased ingestion of clarified butter (known as ghee in the Vedic tradition), as well as the use of sesame oil for massage and other therapies. Ghee has had all solids and impurities removed, and is an especially good source of the type of fatty molecules needed to create cell membranes. Sesame oil is a rich source of polyunsaturated fatty acids, and it also contains potent free radical scavengers.

If cell membranes contain damaged molecules (lipid peroxides and their degenerated descendants), then an influx of ghee and sesame oil could provide intact molecules to replace them.

To study this question, we measured lipid peroxide levels on a number of subjects before, during, and after panchakarma. The results were intriguing. During the week of panchakarma treatments, the blood level of lipid peroxides actually went up. By three months after the treatment, however, the levels were far lower than they had been before treatment began. If you sweep your room, dust will fly temporarily, but soon the room is cleaner than before. Apparently, the ghee, sesame oil and other aspects of panchakarma had loosened lipid peroxides from cell membranes and set them free, circulating in the blood. In the weeks after panchakarma, the body eliminated these circulating lipid peroxide molecules—and the rate at which new ones were being produced apparently declined.

In addition, panchakarma significantly lowered the stress syndrome that creates free radicals. The soothing massages and other relaxing treatments during panchakarma are metabolized into the physiology. Anxiety, as measured by a standard psychological test, declined markedly.

Moreover, the study showed that panchakarma improved several cardiovascular risk factors. VIP (*vasoactive intestinal peptide*), a neuropeptide which dilates the coronary arteries, rose by 80% three months after panchakarma. HDL (High Density Lipoprotein) cholesterol, the "good" (free radical-resistant) cholesterol, rose 75% after three months in those subjects who had original values that were low.

Panchakarma thus seems to be another effective means to rebalance the physiology—and put scavenger and repair mechanisms ahead in their race against free radical damage.

MAHARISHI GANDHARV VED

Sound is an ingestible experience. It can alter the physiology. In fact, sound may be especially potent. Quantum mechanics tells us that the sub-atomic particles and forces that constitute the body are fundamentally wave vibrations. It is not illogical to assume that these wave vibrations could be affected by the wave vibrations of sound. Well-publicized research has shown that music affects the growth of plants, and has also shown significant effects of sound on the human physiology and psychology.

In truth, the fields of music and medicine have been linked throughout the ages. Primitive man used music to ward off evil spirits thought to cause disease. In ancient Greece, the philosophers carried out investigations on music's effect on the body, and music was applied systematically as a curative or preventive modality. It was used to treat insomnia and as an aid to digestion during meals. The Persians and the Hebrews also employed music as therapy for a variety of illnesses, and during the Renaissance, inquiring minds investigated music's influence on breathing, blood pressure, muscular activity, and digestion.[11]

Throughout most of the 20th century, the object-oriented technologies of modern medicine have obscured the traditionally close relationship between music and medicine. Over the last 30 years, however, there has been renewed interest in the use of music as a medical treatment. Music therapy has emerged as a rational discipline supported by extensive research evidence, with professional training and recognized qualifications.[12]

Research on music: Investigations have shown that music has many effects on the human body. One study demonstrated that music can change pulse rate, circulation, and blood pressure.[13] Depending on the type of music played, there can be an increase or decrease in metabolism, internal secretions related to metabolic change, muscular energy, and respiration rate.[14] One study showed specifically that soothing music decreases oxygen consumption and basal metabolic rate, while exciting music increases both.[15] Widespread effects in the body have been demonstrated by another study which showed that different types of music have different effects on gastric motility, electrical conductivity of the skin, pupillary dilation, and muscle contraction.[16]

Music has been utilized specifically as a treatment. A large number of studies have revealed that music can help alleviate acute pain.[17] In fact, music has decreased the need for pain medication and sedatives as much as 30%.[18] Music therapy is now used on a regular basis in the delivery room at the University of Kansas Medical Center in Kansas City—where it routinely lowers the amount of anesthesia needed and shortens the labor period.[19]

Vibrations among the molecules: Recent research has provided a molecular-level explanation for the effect of music—and all types of sound—on the functioning of cells. Cells, subcellular components, and molecules all exhibit characteristic vibrational patterns. DNA structures containing G-C base pairs, for instance, vibrate at a higher frequency than those containing A-T base pairs.[20] Proteins have been measured with specific vibrational frequencies registering one trillion oscillations per second and higher.[21] These vibrations have functional importance. Vibrations of the myoglobin molecule, for example, encourage the movement of oxygen molecules in and out of the molecular structure. Structural vibrations in enzymes also appear to be important at the active site—where substrate molecules are joined or sundered.[22]

Throughout the cell and extending into the extracellular spaces is a skeletal structure which also has characteristic vibrations. In the nucleus, this semi-rigid maze is known as the nuclear matrix. In the cytoplasm, a similar web-like structure is called the cytoskeleton. Outside the cell, it is known as the extracellular matrix.[23] All three components of this matrix system are interconnected, and maintain constant vibrational activity.

The rapid vibrations of this system have mechanical effects in the cell. When molecules such as messenger RNA move in and out of the nucleus, they appear to move down lines of this matrix system, guided by the direction of matrix fibers and motivated by their vibrational energy.[24] Some researchers believe that fluctuations in the vibrational rate moving down the matrix fibers act as a communication system. Even signals from outside the cell can be transmitted through the connecting matrix system all the way to the DNA.[25] Recent studies have also shown that variations in vibrational frequency correlate with various types of cell growth.[26] Cancer cells have a vibrational pattern distinct from all normal cells. [27]

In view of these findings, it is not unreasonable to assume that every cell in the body can respond to changes in vibrational frequency coming from the outside environment. When music soothes the savage beast, it may do so by altering the vibrational pattern in each cell's cellular matrix and DNA.

Music in Maharishi Ayur-Ved: These recent investigations help explain why music of different types plays a central role in Maharishi Ayur-Ved. First, the external vibrations produced by music in the environment almost certainly alter inner vibrations at the molecular level. Second, the melody and rhythmic structure of music is yet another experience to be metabolized through the limbic system—transforming it into a waterfall of neurochemicals and hormones that regenerate the body. Research studies have shown that different types of music have different effects—and masters of the ayurvedic tradition, with sensibilities refined by years of meditation, have conducted a thorough study of these effects of sound on consciousness. The result is a varied pharmacopoeia of music and other uses of sound.

Gandharv Ved: The best known of these is Gandharv Ved, the traditional classical music of India. Gandharv Ved originated thousands of years ago, and even today its basic principles underlie the long and beautiful improvisations by its master musicians.

The doshas can be aggravated or balanced by varying melodies and rhythms. Gandharv Ved is precisely calculated to have a positive effect on dosha balance. In fact, the classical ayurvedic texts list precise times of the day for the playing of different ragas, or melodies. One raga helps create energy and dynamism for activity during the day, another creates restfulness after the evening meal. The music that is right at dawn does not have an ideal effect at noon or midnight.

Maharishi Ayur-Ved emphasizes the importance of these natural cycles of the day (and also the cycle of the seasons—see Behavior below). Listening to Maharishi Gandharv Ved at the right times of the day can smooth the natural transitions and allow the body and mind to function effortlessly, in tune with the 24-hour cycle of natural law. Specific Gandharv Ved ragas are also prescribed in Maharishi Ayur-Ved to balance specific doshas.

Maharishi Gandharv Ved can even be played in a home when no one is there to listen. According to the traditional explanations, the music can have an enlivening and balancing influence within the home even without an audience. Gandharv Ved is considered a powerful tool for the creation of harmony and peacefulness, and it can be used to create this atmosphere in the home.

PRIMORDIAL SOUND

Research has demonstrated that different sounds produce different effects in the physiology. Maharishi Ayur-Ved asserts that particular sounds—*primordial sounds*—have the most positive effect on body and mind. The pronunciation, melody, and rhythmic pattern of these sounds have been preserved as the basic source material of the Vedic tradition—in the Rik Ved and three companion collections: Sam Ved, Yajur Ved, and Atharv Ved. According to Maharishi Ayur-Ved, the sound patterns preserved in these collections reflect the primordial vibrations at the basis of nature.

In the unified field, the self-referral interactions of Rishi (knower), Devata (process of knowing), and Chhandas (known) produce intricate patterns of vibrations. These are the fundamental frequencies said to be at the basis of the physical structure of the universe. These vibrations can be directly cognized within the purified consciousness of enlightened people. Within the field of pure intelligence, the most fundamental vibrations or patterns are heard as *primordial sounds*. This is said to be the deepest level of direct intuition, of subjective knowledge.

Once cognized by enlightened sages, these primordial sounds have been brought out onto the level of human speech. Vedic pandits memorize these sequences, and pass them down from father to son through the generations. According to Maharishi Ayur-Ved, people who listen to these primordial sounds enliven those basic frequencies within their own consciousness. The individual awareness is brought in tune with the first fluctuations of the laws of nature. Because the unified field of natural law is a field of supersymmetry, of perfect balance, Maharishi maintains that this experience brings increased balance to the psychophysiology. Both mind and body metabolize the most basic laws of nature.

Research on primordial sound: At Ohio State we recently tested the effect of these primordial sounds on established cancer cell lines in laboratory culture. Five types of cancer cells were tested (lung, colon, brain, breast, and skin) along with one normal fibroblast cell line. In this type of culture, both cancer cells and fibroblast cells ordinarily grow rapidly (the fibroblasts multiply much more rapidly in cell culture than they do in the human body).

For one set of cell lines, primordial sounds were played—particular selections from Sam Ved. For the other set of cell lines, contrasting sounds were chosen—hard rock music by the band AC/DC. Control cells were grown in an incubator in which no music was played.

The results were striking. Primordial sound significantly decreased the average growth in all cell lines. The results were marked enough that the chance of coincidence was less than five in one thousand. In the presence of hard rock music, the effect went the other way. Growth of the cell lines was significantly increased (with a chance of coincidence less than three in one hundred across all the cell lines), but the effects were not as consistent.[28] The decrease in growth of both cancer cells and normal fibroblasts with Sam Ved is consistent with a balancing effect more in tune with the natural laws of the body. This was a pilot study, and more work is needed, but in this area as well, the effectiveness of Maharishi Ayur-Ved received initial confirmation.

SENSES

Every sense has a direct channel to the brain and consequent effects on the whole physiology. Olfactory cells in the nose, for example, are connected to the hypothalamus. At the same time, the message of a particular aroma is carried to the limbic area of the brain surrounding the hypothalamus, which processes emotions, and to the hippocampus, an area of the brain responsible for memory (that's why certain aromas trigger such vivid memories). The sense of smell is hard-wired directly into the experience-metabolizing switchboard.

The various doshas are each allied with particular senses. Vat, for instance, is predominantly associated with hearing and touch, Pitt with sight, and Kaph with taste and smell. People who are predominantly Vat can be upset by loud noises and are often sensitive to the touch of fabrics. Pitt types, especially if they are fair-haired, can have a hard time in bright sunlight. Kaphs, the earthy type, love the tastes and smells of hearth and home.

Physicians trained in Maharishi Ayur-Ved make use of precise knowledge of sensory stimulation to help their patients ingest particular sensory experiences. Each experience stimulates the brain to produce certain neurochemicals which then communicate with cells throughout the body. In addition to the sound and music therapies already mentioned, Maharishi Ayur-Ved prescribes therapies using touch (various types of massage used to soothe and purify the physiology), smell (Aroma therapy), and sight (Color therapy). Recommendations are based on a person's body type and any dosha imbalances that exist.

NEUROMUSCULAR INTEGRATION

Various positions and motions of the body can not only provide physical exercise, but also feed highly specific experience into the limbic metabolizer. As the body moves and stretches, it stimulates muscles, ligaments and tendons, and even the internal organs. Each aspect of this physiological experience is fed to the brain and limbic system through both the nervous system and molecular messengers. Carefully chosen and correctly performed, such physical activity enlivens mind-body integration.

Maharishi Ayur-Ved uses particular Vedic exercises, including *suryanamaskaras* and *yoga asanas*, to produce enhanced psychophysiological functioning. For healthy people, there are general sets of these exercises which are useful for prevention; for the ill, specific techniques are used—some even for the bedridden.

These exercises stimulate blood flow. Seated poses create stability and proper spinal alignment. Forward bends stimulate digestion, increase the spine's flexibility, and calm the body. Backbends also create spinal flexibility. Inverted poses stimulate the endocrine system and allow for increased circulation. Twisting poses aid digestion and elimination, and tone the spinal column.

Vedic exercises are always done easily and in a relaxed way, with no attempt to push or force. They are not gymnastics, intended to race the body and tire it out. Rather, they are precise movements and poses which both relax and enliven the body, increasing energy rather than exhausting it. According to Maharishi Ayur-Ved, regular practice of these exercises helps produce better health and an ingrained sense of well-being.

Research: Extensive research on yoga asanas has been carried out by scientists in India. The studies have shown that these physical postures are a "meditation for the body." They produce many of the same physiological effects as meditation, including physical relaxation, reduced blood pressure, and increased alpha waves in the brain. Long-term effects include reduced cholesterol levels, biochemical changes indicative of healthier functioning in the autonomic nervous system, and decreased blood sugar during fasting, indicating potential prevention of maturity-onset diabetes.[29] Other studies have shown a wide range of symptomatic benefits, including reduction in overweight, improved eyesight, improved appetite, less need for sleep, improved memory and intellect, reduced incidence of the common cold, and improvement in rheumatoid arthritis.[30]

NEURORESPIRATORY INTEGRATION

Breathing exercises in Maharishi Ayur-Ved are a gentle form of balancing the breath. The generic name for such exercises is *pranayam*. Specific breathing techniques are used for specific illnesses and imbalances, and there are general exercises useful for prevention that all people can employ. Some of these exercises involve alternating the breath from one nostril to the other. According to Maharishi Ayur-Ved, this alternation enlivens alternate hemispheres in the brain. Research has shown that the right hemisphere of the brain is typically more spatial and big-picture in its functioning, while the left hemisphere is more linear and detail-oriented. Pranayam is said to enliven and integrate both hemispheres, leading to a more balanced and efficient mind and body.

Pranayam has also been frequently researched. Studies have shown that it increases lung capacity (which usually decreases with age), and decreases pulse rate and cholesterol. Pranayam has also been shown to improve the reactivity of adrenocortical function, indicating an improved ability to cope with stress, and to improve digestion and liver function.[31] Since yoga asanas and pranayam are frequently practiced in succession, their combined effects have also been researched. One study showed physical benefits, such as improved muscular endurance and delayed fatigue.[32] Another study showed many psychological and mental improvements, including decreased neuroticism, decreased mental fatigue, improved cognitive performance, and improved memory.[33]

DIET

In Maharishi Ayur-Ved, great attention is given to the diet. The body creates itself largely from the molecules presented as food. Because nutrition is so basic, all other preventive and therapeutic approaches are said to be maximally effective only if the diet is also appropriate.

As with all Maharishi Ayur-Ved treatments, the main emphasis in diet is to restore balance to the underlying doshas. The optimal diet is one which tends to restore the individual to a state of balance appropriate to his or her body type. A Pitt type, who is constitutionally "hot," for example, would in general be advised to follow a diet which is cooling. Such dietary recommendations, however, may be modified by any current imbalances (a Pitt type may currently have Vat out of balance and therefore need a Vat-pacifying diet), and by changes in the seasons (see below).

Taste as nutrition: For those familiar with Maharishi Ayur-Ved, one of the most surprising aspects of modern nutrition is that it completely excludes taste as a consideration. Taste, after all, is the primary experience of every food that is eaten. The body eventually metabolizes the molecular constituents of the food, but it first metabolizes the sensory experience of the taste. The taste receptors are exquisitely sensitive; sweet taste can be perceived in a dilution of 1/200; salty, 1/400; sour, 1/130,000; and bitter 1/2,000,000.[34]

According to the principles of Maharishi Ayur-Ved, this sensitivity to taste sends messages that inform the body of the complex biochemical qualities of each food. Research has indicated that molecules act on taste cells in particular areas of the oral cavity to trigger signals transmitted to the brain cortex and the limbic system (including the hypothalamus). When the taste receptors first experience the different taste and textural properties of a meal, an enormous amount of information is delivered throughout the body (primarily through the limbic system), triggering basic metabolic processes. Long before the food is digested, its influence has spread throughout the body. A delicious meal is more than a treat; the taste can be nourishing in itself.

Diet and body type: This taste-mediated influence is individualized by the body type of the person. Hot food metabolized by a hot Pitt physiology produces a multiplier effect, leading to aggravation. Hot food metabolized by a cold Vat type tends to create balance. In Maharishi Ayur-Ved, the influence of each taste is described by its influence on the doshas.

There are six tastes described in the classical ayurvedic texts: sweet, sour, salty, and bitter (all recognized by Western nutritional science), and pungent and astringent (ordinarily overlooked in the West). Pungent foods are hot and spicy. Astringent foods are drying and absorbent (beans, lentils, the tannin in tea). Some common examples of foods in the sweet, sour, and bitter categories are:

Sweet: milk, butter, rice, bread, and pasta

Sour: yogurt, lemon, and cheese

Bitter: spinach, leafy green vegetables, turmeric

All six tastes should be present in every meal, but certain tastes can be emphasized in order to balance an aggravated dosha. The balancing tastes for the three doshas are:

Vat is balanced by salty, sour, and sweet.

Pitt is balanced by bitter, sweet, and astringent.

Kaph is balanced by pungent, bitter, and astringent.

Although taste is a predominant consideration in dietary recommendations, there are six other qualities of food which also influence nutritional needs. These food qualities are heavy and light, oily and dry, hot (spicy or heated) and cold. Some examples are:

Heavy: cheese, yogurt, wheat products

Light: spinach, apples, corn, barley

Oily: dairy products, fatty foods, oils

Dry: barley, corn, potato, beans

Hot: hot food or drink

Cold: cold food or drink

As with taste, these six qualities can be used to balance an aggravated dosha:

Vat is balanced by hot, heavy, and oily.

Pitt is balanced by cold, heavy, and oily.

Kaph is balanced by hot, light, and dry.

Maharishi Ayur-Ved also emphasizes the importance of the manner in which food is eaten. Meals should be taken graciously, in a settled, comfortable atmosphere, sitting down, with good company, at regular times every day. The nervous system and physiology are metabolizing taste as the food is eaten. This happens most effectively when the physiology is calm and the mood is positive. With a rushed, fast-food meal, the body primarily metabolizes stress.

The main meal should be at lunch time, since Pitt is highest then, with only a light dinner. Digestion is aided by sitting easily for five minutes after finishing the meal.

BEHAVIOR

There is increasing interest in behavioral medicine. Research is making it clear that people can work themselves sick, or predispose illness by not getting enough sleep.

Although modern medicine has not yet developed a comprehensive theory of healthy behavior, such a theory is integral to Maharishi Ayur-Ved. There are regular cycles in the functioning of natural law—daily rhythms and seasonal rhythms. By living in accord with these natural cycles, we can work with, rather than against, the forces of natural law. For example, activity is naturally supported during daylight hours, when the sun warms the atmosphere and our molecules naturally tend to jostle more easily through their chemical reactions. To rise with the sun and sleep in the night is to live in accord with the laws of nature. No one is a "night person" by nature—although aggravation of Vat, the dosha of movement, can keep us running at all hours. Maharishi Ayur-Ved gives simple recommendations regarding when to arise and retire, when to exercise and meditate, when to work and eat.

From season to season, there are also simple recommendations for adjusting the diet and aligning with the weather. This seasonal emphasis has recently received scientific validation from the new field of chronobiology. Over the last fifteen years, a number of illnesses have been studied to see if their occurrence varies over the course of the year. One study has found that heart disease and respiratory disease are greatest in mid-winter and least in the summer.[35] Asthma and bronchitis reach their lowest levels in mid-summer. In some people, peptic ulcers occur most frequently in the spring; for others in the fall.

Metabolizing the seasons: In Maharishi Ayur-Ved, changes in the seasons are understood to create fundamental shifts in biochemistry and metabolic style. Variations in sunlight, heat, cold, wind, and moisture are metabolized by the body. Variations in nature are mirrored by variations in the human physiology. Though the body responds continually and instantaneously to every subtle fluctuation in its environment, the changes become significant as the passing seasons bring long-term trends in the weather. In windy and cold weather, for example, Vat types (who are light and cold) can be adversely affected. Their Vat dosha becomes imbalanced. The period during which the seasons change, producing major changes in the body, is considered to be a time of maximum vulnerability to disease. Since ulcer is considered to be a Pitt disorder, it is no surprise that it occurs principally at the transition times into and out of the hot summer season.

The seasons themselves are classified according to the doshas. In the ayurvedic framework, the year is divided into three seasons instead of the usual four experienced in Northern climate zones. Spring is considered Kaph season, mid-March to mid-June. Spring fever is explained by an aggravation of the slow, heavy Kaph dosha. Summer and early autumn are the Pitt season, mid-June to mid-October. Autumn and winter are the Vat season, mid-October to mid-March. The divisions on the calendar are only guidelines, however. In a subtropical area such as Florida, Pitt conditions prevail throughout most of the year, with only a brief Vat period (December–January) and Kaph period (February–March).

It is no surprise that Maharishi Ayur-Ved recommends that diet be adjusted according to season. It is not a good idea to eat heavy, sweet foods in the spring, for example, when excess Kaph may already be weighing one down. A Kaph type must be especially careful in the spring to eat foods that balance Kaph. Vat and Pitt types should also favor foods that balance Kaph, but not to as great an extent. The same principles hold true in Pitt and Vat seasons.

Adjusting our behavior to daily and seasonal routines puts the body and mind in tune with the functioning of the laws of nature. By promoting behavior in accord with natural law, these routines maintain the integrity of key biological rhythms. In the classical texts of ayurveda, this aspect of life is given great importance for promoting good health and longevity.

PSYCHOPHYSIOLOGICAL INTEGRATION

Conventional psychology and medicine concentrate on abnormal and disease states. They have little to say about the nature of good health and good feelings. Maharishi Ayur-Ved, on the other hand, begins with the concept of ideal health— mind and body perfectly balanced and integrated. Such a state of perfect health produces an inner experience of exhilaration and joy, an experience which, in its fulfilled state, is referred to as bliss.

Each dosha expresses a different aspect of this inner happiness or bliss:

Vat: exhilarating, alert, cheerful, optimistic

Pitt: content, joyous, chivalrous, pleasant, clear-minded

Kaph: steady, strong, forgiving, courageous, generous, affectionate, serene

Most people feel such emotions only at peak moments in their lives. Maharishi Ayur-Ved offers a particular technique—the Psychophysiological Integration technique—

which cultures this rich inner experience called bliss. The Vedic tradition indicates that feelings of intense happiness and bliss are intimately connected with the free flow of intelligence throughout the body and mind. Techniques for bliss-development thus improve both physical and mental health.

EMOTIONS

Many research studies have shown that the emotional state of a patient directly influences the ability to get well. One much-publicized study indicates that, among men who have had serious heart attacks, those who believe their wives love them have a much better chance of full recovery. As we have mentioned, anger correlates with heart disease. Depression is well-known to weaken the immune system and encourage illness of all types.

Many of the approaches of Maharishi Ayur-Ved specifically work to enhance emotional well-being—especially Transcendental Meditation and the Psychophysiological Integration (or "bliss") technique. Doctors trained in Maharishi Ayur-Ved explain to their patients the value of emotions in health and encourage them to take part in programs that can enhance their emotional well-being. We have seen that emotions registered in the limbic region of the brain intimately affect the functioning of the hypothalamus and pituitary. By living a life that cultures the finest feeling levels deep within, by enhancing feelings of inner peace, satisfaction, happiness and, ultimately, bliss, we encourage the body and brain to produce those chemicals that strengthen and sustain physical health. In many ways, happiness *is* health.

INTELLECT

Maharishi Ayur-Ved indicates that Pragya-aparadh, the mistake of the intellect, is integral to both physical creation and the human physiology (see Chapter Eight). It is the intellect which discriminates knower, knowing, and known in the undifferentiated unity of pure consciousness. When the intellect gets lost in the interplay of the three—and forgets the unity, the Samhita—that is Pragya-aparadh.

This intellectual mistake creates a disruptive influence in the psychophysiology. Matter is based on mind. The body is based on the unified field of pure intelligence. When this fundamental fact is lost to the awareness, then mind and body are dis-integrated. The focus then is only on the physical body and its myriad details, and the natural healing power that flows from intelligence to the body is not encouraged.

For this reason, Maharishi Ayur-Ved provides a teaching program for each patient. The goal of this program is to allow patients to remember their own nature, to reconnect their individual life with its unified source in pure consciousness. This intellectual understanding puts the attention back on wholeness, on mind *and* body, on unity *and* diversity. Attention on the totality of life is necessary for perfect health.

LANGUAGE

Language and speech directly transform the physical body. They are manifestations of pure intelligence expressed through the physiology. When a word or sentence comes to mind, particular fluctuations or vibrations appear in the brain, move through the nervous system, and appear as physical action. When a speaker is animated, the entire body comes into play—helping convey both meaning and feeling. Thus, the act of speech can enliven the entire physiology with patterns of underlying intelligence.

Which patterns of intelligence will become lively? The question is vital. Maharishi Ayur-Ved emphasizes the importance of language in the creation of perfect health. It recommends the use of speech that is inspiring and uplifting, speech that unites, speech that is nourishing to life. It is especially important to culture the ability to speak only truth—but to speak the truth that is sweet, truth that spreads only good feelings. The physician is encouraged to develop and apply these principles of health-giving speech, but it is equally important for the patient to do so. The use of language is an especially intimate experience, and like all experiences it is metabolized in the psychophysiology. To a significant degree, we create our health through language.

Sanskrit and health: In this regard, one language is considered to be of particular importance. This is Sanskrit, the language of the Vedic tradition. Sanskrit is the oldest language in the Indo-European family, and most Western languages can be traced back to roots in Sanskrit. Where did Sanskrit originate? We have seen that Maharishi Ayur-Ved makes use of primordial sounds. These are said to be subtle fluctuations in the field of intelligence which have been heard, or cognized, by enlightened sages. When a person of sufficiently purified consciousness hears these first murmurings of intelligence interacting with itself, that person is hearing the sounds of the Sanskrit language. Maharishi explains that Sanskrit was not invented but, like mathematical truths, cognized fully-formed in subtle levels of the mind. Because these sounds are said to represent the most basic patterns of natural law underlying the diversity of the manifest universe, Sanskrit is referred to as the "language of nature."

For this reason, it is held that speaking the sounds of the Sanskrit language can have health-generating effects. In this case, it is the sounds, the vibrations, not the word meanings, which are important. Even without understanding the words, a patient can bring both mind and body into attunement with natural law simply by reciting the sounds of the language of nature. Maharishi Ayur-Ved indicates that the wave forms of Sanskrit are so fundamental that, as they move from the mind to the brain and throughout the body, they rebalance the psychophysiology. Perfect speech helps create perfect health.

PULSE DIAGNOSIS

In addition to the use of standard patient histories and physical examinations, doctors trained in Maharishi Ayur-Ved use a unique system of pulse diagnosis. The master vaidyas of ayurveda have always maintained that the subtle fluctuations of the body's underlying field of intelligence are reflected in a person's pulse. By placing three fingers on the pulse in the wrist, a physician can evaluate imbalances in the doshas. The "deep" pulse, evaluated with a firm touch on the wrist, reflects a person's basic body type. More superficial fluctuations in the pulse, felt with a lighter touch, give knowledge about current imbalances.

This knowledge allows physicians to prescribe individualized health care programs for both prevention and treatment of disease. Pulse diagnosis is especially valuable for determining early stages of dosha imbalance, when there may be no outward symptoms. By correcting the imbalance immediately with mild therapies, overt disease can be prevented.

It is possible to learn how to monitor your own pulse. By checking the pulse at different times of the day, you can watch the temporary rise and fall of the doshas and gain an understanding of which activities are most likely to cause imbalances or help regain balance. Just as a switchboard has access to all the telephone lines in the building, so pulse diagnosis gives access to activity everywhere in the body.

MAHARISHI JYOTISH

Quantum physics has discovered that all of nature is deeply interconnected. From one end of the universe to the other, all protons and electrons, all galaxies and stars, are simply fluctuations in the unbounded, unified field of pure intelligence. Einstein's theory of relativity showed that space and time are part of one continuum—space-time. In relativity theory, moreover, measurements of the "objective" space-time continuum are inseparably linked to the state of the observer (the subject, the knower). The length of a ruler, for example, depends on the relative speed of the person observing it.

Quantum mechanical investigations have shown the same deep relationship of subject and object, observer and observed (see Chapter Seven). Recent investigations have also demonstrated that any two sub-atomic "particles," once they have interacted, are permanently and instantaneously connected across even an infinite distance. If you use an electromagnetic field to flip one particle over, the other will flip at the same time, no matter how far away, and with no material connection between the two. To many physicists, these deep interconnections seem a central element of physical creation. Nothing exists on its own, not even the finest fluctuation. In the words of University of California physicist H.P. Stapp: "An elementary particle is not an independently existing unanalyzable entity. It is, in essence, a set of relationships that reach outward to other things."[36]

These deep relationships throughout creation—including connections between the objective world and the human mind —have long been understood and utilized in the tradition of ayurveda. This branch of knowledge is known as Jyotish. Trained Maharishi Jyotish experts use precise mathematical calculations to take into account important aspects of the environment, including planets and stars. These calculations are said to yield information about the health of an individual. Most importantly, this information can be used to predict health problems coming in the future. Maharishi frequently quotes a central Vedic text: *Heyam dukham anagatam* ("Avert the danger that has not yet come"). In Maharishi Ayur-Ved, Jyotish is used to foresee dangers so proper preventive measures can be employed in time.

MAHARISHI YAGYA

Yagya (YAHG-yuh) is based on the same principle as primordial sound and the recitation of Sanskrit. Sequences of sounds cognized by enlightened seers amount to a blueprint of the most basic laws of nature, "DNA" for the universe. Physicists speak of the "cosmic code," the mathematically describable laws of nature that structure creation. In Maharishi's explanation, the complex sound patterns in Rik Ved and other central Vedic texts *are* this cosmic code. Information is carried by pronunciation, pitch, sequence, and rhythmic pattern. Every law of nature has its own unique pattern.

Maharishi Yagya involves groups of trained experts in the field of Vedic knowledge—known as pandits (PUN-dits)—who perform particular sequences from these Vedic collections. The performance is said to enliven the particular laws of nature that correspond to the selections. This brings balance to the environment as a whole. Yagyas can be performed for individuals, groups, nations, and the world as a whole. Choice of the particular Yagya to be performed is often based on the calculations of Jyotish—so that Yagyas can be used to correct imbalances that have not yet manifested. The relative impact of the Yagya is proportional to both the number of, and the purity of the awareness of, the pandits who perform it.

ENVIRONMENT

Everyone knows that air and water pollution have become major causes of human disease. In addition, the *sick building syndrome* is now a recognized ailment of modern society. Builders have used increasingly toxic materials—including dyes, paints, and glues in wood products, carpets, and other materials. At the same time, buildings have been deliberately constructed to seal them tight, so air conditioning and heating can work efficiently. The result is that toxic fumes are trapped inside. There is also growing concern about sources of low-level electromagnetic fields, such as high voltage power lines, video display terminals, and electric blankets. It is suspected that, over time, these electromagnetic fields may be detrimental to our health. In other words, our homes and offices can make us sick.

In addition, recent research studies have shown that overcrowding in any environment also leads to problems with psychological health, problems that soon spill over into physical health. Taken together, these facts add to the notion that we have constructed a civilization that is dangerous to our health. Using modern technologies without regard to their dangers, we have built not just sick buildings, but a sick society. In a sense that is much too real, our environment is a pathogen.

Maharishi Ayur-Ved addresses these environmental concerns. Through knowledge of Sthapatya Ved, the Vedic science of construction, Maharishi Ayur-Ved makes a series of specific recommendations about living and working environments. Sthapatya Ved offers construction in tune with the laws of nature. It recommends non-toxic materials, for example, and it arranges the rooms in a house with respect to the path of the sun during the course of the day, so energy levels are correct for each type of activity. The informing principle behind Sthapatya Ved is that our lives can never be maximally healthy until we live in structures that are themselves healthy.

WORLD HEALTH/WORLD PEACE

Some of the most convincing research on Maharishi Ayur-Ved has been conducted on the most far-reaching of all Maharishi Ayur-Ved programs. Meditation can change the world around us. A famous phrase from the Vedic literature reads, *Tat sannidhau vairatyagah* ("In the vicinity of the settled mind, hostile tendencies fall away"). Now, more than forty separate scientific studies have shown that practiced meditation experts actually can create a statistically measurable influence of harmony and peace in their environment.

These studies show that, whenever attendance increases at an assembly of experts in Transcendental Meditation and the TM-Sidhi program, crime decreases, traffic accidents go down, and open warfare (if it is present) declines. The incidence of infectious disease has also been shown to fall. At the same time, the economy begins to improve—as measured by unemployment, inflation, stock market activity, gross domestic product, and other statistics.

At first, it might seem impossible that a group of meditators in one spot could reduce accidents and illness hundreds of miles away. In fact, this follows naturally if consciousness is indeed a field. Any field in nature can support radiating waves that create *field effects* and *action at a distance*. A television station can radiate invisible, non-material waves through the underlying electromagnetic field. The result is a TV picture in your living room.

We have seen strong reasons to suppose that consciousness, like every other aspect of nature, is also an unbounded field. Now, research on "the group dynamics of consciousness" known as the Maharishi Effect provides clear evidence that consciousness does indeed have a field-like nature. It supports field effects that radiate even halfway around the world, producing action at a distance—reduced crime and violence, and improved economic growth.

Expert acceptance: These signs of social health have been clearly indicated in a number of research studies that have been carefully examined by independent experts, then accepted for publication in academic journals. Scholars have been especially impressed by tight correlations over long periods of time. Whenever the attendance at a Transcendental Meditation assembly rises, the social statistics improve. If the attendance falls again, the statistics regress. Changes in the attendance at the meditation assembly commonly occur just *before* changes in the social statistics—and the cause must obviously occur before the effect. These correlations have often gone on for many years.

The statistical power of the studies has impressed many independent academic experts. Says Raymond Russ, Ph.D., Professor of Psychology at the University of Maine, and editor of the *Journal of Mind and Behavior* (which has published two of the studies), "The hypothesis definitely raised some eyebrows among our reviewers. But the statistical work was sound. The numbers were there. . . . When you can statistically control for as many variables as these studies do, it makes the results more convincing."[37]

Ted Robert Gurr, Ph.D., Professor of Government and Politics at the University of Maryland, is one of the most respected scholars in the field of conflict analysis. He says, "In the studies that I have examined on the impact of the Maharishi Effect on conflict I can find no methodological flaws, and the findings have been consistent across a large number of replications in many different geographical and conflictual situations."[38]

David Edwards, Ph.D., Professor of Government at the University of Texas at Austin, has commented on this research at academic conferences. He says, "I think the claim can plausibly be made that the potential impact of this research exceeds that of any other ongoing social or psychological research program. The research has survived a broader array of statistical tests than most research in the field of conflict resolution. I think this work, and the theory that informs it, deserves the most serious consideration by academics and policy makers alike."[39]

According to this research evidence, the profound understanding of consciousness provided by Maharishi Ayur-Ved has produced a scientific discovery of immeasurable impact. Repreated studies indicate that groups of meditators can transform whole societies. Age-old social ills such as crime and warfare, social tension and economic malfunction, can finally be addressed with a scientifically validated technology.

Even for our own individual health, this discovery is vital. The stress and tension of modern societies mass produce free radicals in every individual in society. The fear of crime on the streets, the reality of hostility in the office, the uncertainty of the nation's economic future—all these social ailments are metabolized by every citizen. Social ills create physical ills. For each of us to enjoy ideal health, we must not only focus on our own mind and body. We must also transform the society around us. Maharishi Ayur-Ved addresses this problem with a systematic technique.

MAHARISHI AYUR-VED AT A GLANCE

As this brief survey has indicated, Maharishi Ayur-Ved is a comprehensive and integrated system of natural health care. From the standpoint of modern medicine, its twenty approaches are without doubt innovative and unusual. But modern medicine clearly needs assistance, and only a new seed can yield a new crop.

As I became familiar with these various approaches over the last decade, two things struck me most forcibly. First was the detailed and ingenious ways in which Maharishi Ayur-Ved addressed the mind and body to produce subtle transformations. This body of knowledge does not appear to be incomplete and experimental, feeling its way through trial and error toward effective technologies. It appears rather to be a sophisticated and mature approach, taking into account realities of the human psychophysiology which modern science is only beginning to glimpse.

Second, whenever the various approaches of Maharishi Ayur-Ved have been tested scientifically, the results have been uniformly positive. On the most fundamental issue of modern medical science—free radicals and their damage—the objective benefits demonstrated for Maharishi Ayur-Ved have been the most impressive.

Maharishi Ayur-Ved appears in modern societies as a completely new approach to the health of both body and mind. It is constructed on the consciousness paradigm—the theory that consciousness is primary, and that matter is derived from consciousness. It is a health care system intended to restore the connection between consciousness and physiology, between mind and body, and to therefore correct physiological imbalances at their source. It is prevention-oriented, free of serious side effects, and, according to the research evidence, unprecedentedly effective.

In fact, the very success of this integrated system of natural health care raises intriguing questions. If we grant that human health can be dramatically enhanced, conundrums still exist. Are health and long life ends in themselves, for example? Or is there a deeper purpose behind the search for perfect health?

It is time to assess the implications of the discoveries set forth in this book.

Notes

1. Ironson G, et al, *Am J Cardiol* 70(1992): 281-5; Musante L, et al, *Behav Med* 18(1992): 21-6; Barefoot JC, et al, *Psychosom Med* 45(1983): 59-63

2. Schneider R, et al, presented at the Eighth World Congress of the International College of Psychosomatic Medicine, Chicago, September, 1985

3. *Shushrut Samhita*, Sutrasthanam, Chapter 24, 19 (Chaukhambha Orientalis, New Delhi)

4. Klein DB, *The Concept of Consciousness: A Survey* (University of Nebraska Press, Lincoln, 1984), quoted in front matter

5. Oates RM Jr., *Celebrating the Dawn* (G.P. Putnam's Sons, New York, 1976), pp. 186-7

6. Ibid, p. 191

7. Maharishi Mahesh Yogi, *Life Supported by Natural Law* (Age of Enlightenment Press, Washington, DC, 1986), p. 25

8. Ibid, p. 29-30

9. Ibid, pp. 111-2

10. Ibid, pp. 46-7

11. Alvin J, *Music Therapy* (John Baker Publishers, Ltd., London, 1966); Cook JD, *Cancer Nurs* 9(1986): 23-8; Cook JD, *Nurs Forum* 20(1981): 252-66

12. Randall T, *JAMA* 266(1991): 1323-9; Cook, *Cancer* (see note 11); Alvin J, *Physiotherapy* 64(1978): 77-9

13. MacClelland DC, *AORN J* 29(1979): 252-60

14. Ibid

15. Ibid; Cook, *Cancer* (see note 11)

16. Bruya MA, Severtsen B, *J Neurosurg Nurs* 16(1984): 96-100

17. Cook, *Cancer*; (see note 11); Munro S, Mount B, *Can Med Assoc J* 119(1978): 1029-34; Owens MK, Ehrenreich D, *Holist Nurs Pract* 6(1991): 24-31; O'Sullivan RJ, *Intens Care Nurs* 7(1991):160-3; Cook, *Nurs* (see note 11)

18. Owens, *Holist* (see note 17); Cook, *Cancer* (see note 11)

19. Cook, *Nurs* (see note 11)

20. Chou K-C, *Biochem J* 221(1984): 27-31

21. Chou K-C, *Biochem J* 209(1983): 573-80

22. Karplus M, McCammon JA, *Sci Am* 254(4)(1986): 42-51; Sitter AJ, et al, *Biochim Biophys Acta* 828(1985): 229-35

23. Isaacs JT, et al, *Prog Clin Biol Res* 75A(1981): 1-24; Shaper JH, et al, *Advances Enz Reg* 17(1978): 213-48

24. Lawrence JB, et al, *Cell* 57(1989): 493-502; Xing Y, Lawrence JB, *J Cell Biol* 109(1989): 315a (Abstract)

25. Pienta KJ, Coffey DS, *Medical Hypotheses* 34(1991): 88-95

26. Myrdal SE, Auersperg N, *J Cell Biol* 102(1986): 1224

27. Partin AW, et al, *Cancer Res* 48(1988): 6050-3; Mohler JL, et al, *J Urol* 138(1987): 168

28. Stephens RE, et al, *J Fed Am Soc Exper Biol*, 6(1992): A1934 (Abstract)

29. Joseph S, et al, *Ind J Med Res* 74(1981): 120-4

30. *Studies on the Efficacy of Yoga in the Promotion and Maintenance of Normal Health Aspects in Yoga Trainees*, Central Council for Research in Yog and Naturopathy, Ministry of Health and Family Welfare, Government of India (1989), p. 14

31. Udupa KN, et al, *Ind J Med Res* 63(8)(1975): 1062-5; Nayar HS, et al, *Ind J Med Res* 63(10)(1975): 1369-76

32. Ray US, et al, *Ind J Med Res* 83(1986): 343-8

33. Udupa KN, et al, *Ind J Med Res* 61(2)(1973): 237-44

34. Ackerman D, *A Natural History of the Senses* (Random House, New York, 1990), pp. 127-72

35. Hayes DK, et al, eds. "Chronobiology: Its Role in Clinical Medicine, General Biology, and Agriculture" in *Progress in Clinical and Biological Research, Vol 341, A & B*, (Wiley-Liss, New York, 1990)

36. Davies P, *Superforce: The Search for a Grand Unified Theory of Nature* (Touchstone, Simon & Schuster, New York, 1984), p. 49

37. Raymond Russ, Ph.D., Professor of Psychology at the University of Maine, and editor of the *Journal of Mind and Behavior*, personal communication (May 1992)

38. Ted Robert Gurr, Ph.D., Professor of Government and Politics at the University of Maryland, personal communication (May 1992)

39. David Edwards, Ph.D., and Professor of Government at the University of Texas at Austin, personal communication (May 1992)

Toward a
Disease-Free Society

A new era for human life and health has begun. I am convinced this is true. The research has been carried out and the evidence is in the academic journals.

Until now, life promised illness and aging at a pre-set pace. By watching our parents and grandparents, and the elder generations in the society around us, we could predict with disturbing precision the arc of life we ourselves could expect. We could predict, at least on average, the onset of serious disease. We could predict the rate of increasing dysfunction. We could predict the approximate time when accumulated physiological damage would render the body altogether unusable.

Fortunately, that data no longer applies. Generations in the past were worn down by free radical attack—and never even knew their enemy. Now the molecular world is well understood. The rampant destruction caused by oxy radicals and ROS has been thoroughly documented. Without this knowledge, the rate and severity of aging and disease might have seemed an unavoidable aspect of human nature, and our physiological decline inevitable and out of our control. But problems caused by darkness disappear in the light. Problems caused by ignorance vanish in the light of knowledge.

In the late nineteenth century, Pasteur's discovery of one-celled microbes led to rapid reduction of infectious disease. In the late twentieth century, the free radical paradigm, combined with effective programs to counter free radicals, promises to dramatically reduce degenerative disease. Reducing the oxidative stress caused by free radicals also provides backup protection to further reduce infectious disease—by strengthening the effectiveness of the immune system.

We now have curative and preventive leverage on both infectious and degenerative diseases. Hundreds of published scientific studies indicate that it may actually be possible for every nation to make rapid progress toward the goal first enunciated by Maharishi: The creation of a disease-free society.

VALIDATING MIND-BODY MEDICINE

For millennia, sages in the ancient Vedic tradition of knowledge have extolled the virtues of meditation. They have lauded the healing powers of simple herbal formulations. They have told all who would listen that human life can be transformed, that mind and body can be refined, that problems and suffering can be left behind.

Now, for the first time, objective evidence indicates that their assertions are true. Some of the smallest constituents of the "material" world—oxy radicals and ROS—have helped us understand the value of health care based on consciousness.

Just as the free radical challenge has helped validate Maharishi Ayur-Ved, so Maharishi Ayur-Ved has helped validate the mind-body approach to medicine. Psychoneuroimmunology had already pieced together the hard wiring that connects mind and body. It had established the limbic-hypothalamus-pituitary nexus, where thoughts and feelings turn into regulatory molecules. It had traced the biochemical conversation between the hypothalamus and the immune system, the two-way communication that keeps the mind and the physical defenses on the same page. What mind-body medicine had failed to do was provide practical applications that took advantage of these discoveries.

The rich and varied approaches of Maharishi Ayur-Ved have filled this vacuum. There is no longer any doubt as to whether mind-body medicine can be effective—when the technologies used are profound. Transcendental Meditation, for example, reduces stress; reduced stress reduces catecholamines; reduced catecholamines reduces free radicals; reduced free radicals reduces molecular damage in the cells of the body; reduced molecular damage reduces disease; reduced disease reduces hospitalization; reduced hospitalization reduces health care costs. From an abstract mental experience to a concrete, hard cash measure, every step in the chain is now established through objective science.

CAN IT BE TRUE?

For some people, these prospects may seem too good to be true. I've had scientists review the research on Maharishi Amrit Kalash and Transcendental Meditation and tell me it just *can't* be true. How can a mixture of flowers and roots and fruits possibly affect cancer, heart disease, inflammatory diseases, the immune system, pollutants, aging, and psychological mood? How can sitting quietly with the eyes closed reduce health care costs by more than 50% all by itself? Medical researchers have often spent long years looking for a single cure for a single disease—not infrequently in vain. Nothing in their background has prepared them for simple approaches that counter most major diseases—and apparently offer increased preventive protection against them all.

I can empathize with these feelings because I have had them. As I mentioned in the Introduction, I was quite reluctant at first to get involved in research on a chemically mysterious selection of herbs and fruits. My first-hand experience, however, has made all the difference. When you watch experiments unfold day after day, when you supervise the data analysis and confront the results, a lifetime of preconceptions can be washed away.

In fact, I firmly believe that if MAK were a drug, if it were the latest discovery from a major pharmaceutical company, it would be the most widely-publicized miracle cure in the medical world right now. Similarly, it seems to me that if Transcendental Meditation were a machine, an electromagnetic device that stabilized the autonomic nervous system in just 20 minutes twice a day—producing all the health benefits that Transcendental Meditation has demonstrated so far—millions of units would sell every year.

What accounts for the delay in acceptance? With Americans more interested in their personal health than ever before, and our national health care system in both functional and financial crisis, what is preventing scientists, government leaders, and the general public from immediately adopting these proven techniques from the ancient ayurvedic tradition? This book is written with the intention of putting a stop to the free radical destruction of individual health and national budgets. From this perspective, these questions are important. It is pointless for scientists to make significant discoveries if they are not put to use.

BEYOND SIMPLISTIC EXPLANATIONS

I'm sure one reason for the delay is simply cultural discomfort. Every nation has its own traditions and its own pride. New ideas coming from the far side of the world, from an ancient tradition largely unfamiliar, are always more difficult to accept.

It's also true that the nature of the Maharishi Ayur-Ved health care approach is challenging to the world view of modern science. Confronting Maharishi Amrit Kalash specifically, I know that some research scientists are concerned about the complex formulation. They know, in a formula with thousands of molecular types, they will never be able to accurately identify which components produce which benefits. They will never be able to discover all the chemical balances that prevent side effects. Dealing with Transcendental Meditation, the challenge is similar. Research has clearly shown that the Transcendental Meditation technique does not reduce to the active ingredient of relaxation—and scientists typically have no experience with more subtle explanations involving higher states of consciousness. They aren't familiar with the concept of a fourth state of consciousness. They aren't used to the idea that deep inner experience within the mind can produce profound changes in the body.

If we are honest with ourselves as medical investigators, however, we have to admit that even with the most common drugs, our laboratory experiments frequently fail to deliver us clear explanations for effectiveness. The truth is, for long decades we had no idea even how aspirin works. We chase after mechanical explanations, and find some. But much of our medical pharmacopoeia is, in essence, a black box. It works, but we don't know how. If effective drugs often evade clear explanation, why should we worry if effective herbal formulations do so as well?

THE ECONOMIC BARRIER

Even if scientists learn to accept approaches that don't fit easily within their preconceptions, I believe there is one other impediment to rapid acceptance of the Maharishi Ayur-Ved approaches. The main engine for social change in modern industrial societies is the profit motive. The collapse of the communist world has only reinforced our confidence in the free enterprise system, where millions of individuals, making decisions in their own self-interest, are the drivers of economic progress. If an idea is useful, we tend to believe, it will be picked up and packaged solely due to the profit motive.

With ayurvedic approaches, however, we have to realize that established entities in the health care field face severe problems. For example, pharmaceutical companies need something they can patent. To them, an active ingredient is not simply a comfortable fit with their established world view. An active ingredient is vital to their economic success. Such a company needs an isolated molecule that it discovered, or synthesized, and can claim exclusive credit for. No company, however, can claim the credit for whole plants. You can't patent an orange. The credit for the creation of the plant kingdom clearly goes somewhere else. This means that natural herbal supplements can't be patented, protected, and marketed by a single company, the way artificial drugs can. Maharishi Amrit Kalash not only eludes the reductionist approach of modern science. It also eludes the financial structure of modern medicine.

The Transcendental Meditation technique also resists the reductionist approach. It is from an ancient tradition with roots in life lived in higher states of consciousness. It requires teachers that have been trained in all the subtleties of the inner experiences people have as they learn the technique—knowledge only available in the ancient Vedic tradition. Research has shown that alternative techniques do not have the same effect.

For reasons such as these, we now see in modern societies a mounting clash between modern medicine and natural medicine. Although the current health care approaches are clearly insufficient, established medical institutions struggle against natural alternatives. In spite of this, according to an article published in the *New England Journal of Medicine* in January of 1993, one out of every three individuals in the U.S. seek alternative approaches for health care problems. There is an increasing awareness and acceptance of alternative health care by the society as a whole. In fact, the United States Congress has recently mandated the National Institutes of Health to begin a systematic investigation of alternative health care.

CALLING FOOD DRUGS

Regulatory bodies in the government, on the other hand, have recently tended to respond to lobbying from large institutions in their field. An instructive example has been the federal Food and Drug Administration. In the last decade, research on free radicals has finally shown conclusively that certain vitamins, nutrients, and natural herbal food supplements can have markedly beneficial effects on health. Just as this research has begun to gain wide attention, the FDA has suddenly announced that it intends to tightly regulate the sale of vitamins—and to block the sale of most medicinal herbs altogether. The stated reason is safety. A handful of instances of dangerous side effects have been cited—most from impure preparation. For this reason, the FDA reports, it is proposing that vitamins in large doses and herbs in any dose should be unavailable to the public until they go through the same testing requirements that drugs undergo.

This proposal has received wide publicity, and many researchers have criticized it sharply. They point out that artificial drugs have amply proven that they need careful testing, while herbal medicines have been used safely for thousands of years. They point out that the few instances of problems with vitamins and herbs cited by the FDA pale into insignificance compared to the problems caused over recent decades by artificial drugs that have successfully completed FDA requirements. They point out that the American Cancer Society says many vegetables prevent cancer, yet no one suggests that broccoli or Brussels sprouts be regulated. They point out that no one will be able to afford to pay millions of dollars for FDA testing on natural substances that can then be sold on street corners by anyone who so desires. They point out that, if the new regulations go into effect, Americans will be able to freely buy cigarettes (which kill 400,000 people a year); they will be able to freely buy alcohol (which destroys hundreds of thousands of lives and families every year); they will be able to freely buy automatic pistols and assault rifles; but they won't be able to buy Sleepy Time tea. Most significantly, they point out that if Americans are denied access to vitamins and herbal supplements (which can, among other things, slow the destruction caused by free radicals), they will be condemned to earlier illness and the need to use modern medicine, including artificial drugs.

In fact, some observers maintain that the FDA suggestions are, in effect, an act of war by one system of medicine upon another. If the FDA can succeed in imposing the rules of modern medicine upon the approaches of natural medicine, it is possible that only modern medicine will remain. The financial hurdles required to pass FDA testing requirements could mean that natural medicine will simply disappear.

I mention these considerations because they directly affect the health of people in our society. Overcoming free radicals is not simply a matter of scientific investigation. It is also a complex cultural, political, and economic question.

In any event, at this stage of the research on MAK and Transcendental Meditation, I know what my attitude has become. It is completely pragmatic. If it works, use it.

THE SIDE BENEFITS OF HEALTH

The more quickly we take advantage of this consciousness-based approach to mental and physical health, moreover, the more quickly we will gain the advantage of significant side *benefits*. At the beginning, our goal may be just a few more years of healthy, happy living. But the research evidence indicates that, by pursuing good health through a consciousness-based system of natural medicine, we gain rapid mental and psychological growth as well. For the individual, therefore, pursuit of the best free radical defense leads to growth toward a higher quality of life.

In the Vedic tradition, the possibility of such evolution of consciousness is understood. The four great aims of life are said to be artha (wealth), dharma (righteousness), kama (enjoyment), and moksha (enlightenment). Modern bumper stickers say, "He who dies with the most toys wins." But the Vedic tradition has always understood that material success in life (wealth and enjoyment) must be balanced with moral rectitude and the development of higher states of consciousness.

Such an integrated life depends on a high quality of health—both physical and mental. If the body is weak and sluggish, or if the mind is dull and cloudy, success is elusive on any level. If the body is vital and energetic, and if the mind is lively and clear, then every aspect of life can be pursued successfully. This is the purpose of Maharishi Ayur-Ved. By taking a comprehensive and integrated approach that refines both physiology and consciousness, Maharishi Ayur-Ved aims not just for a healthy body but for a healthy life.

BOOSTING CREATIVITY

What's more, just like individuals, whole societies will also enjoy side benefits from a prevention-oriented system of natural health care that actually works. Every society in the world is seeking much more rapid economic growth. And in the Information Age, economists agree, the most important economic resource of any nation is the quality of consciousness available in the work force. Riches are created by intelligence and creativity. Even a resource-poor nation like Japan can rise to economic leadership on sheer brainpower.

We have seen that Maharishi Ayur-Ved provides food supplements that not only control free radicals, but also stimulate brain functioning and increase intelligence and psychological well-being. We have seen that Transcendental Meditation not only reduces stress, but also increases intelligence, creativity, and self-confidence. With widespread use of the consciousness-based programs of Maharishi Ayur-Ved, not only would health care costs fall dramatically. It also appears that every economy would gain a major boost from a systematic upgrade of its most important resource—the consciousness of its people.

THE IMPLICATIONS OF LONGEVITY

The research evidence on free radical control is already strong enough to have provoked among some people a philosophical discussion on the implications of longevity. As life span begins to lengthen, this will only emphasize the oldest of moral dilemmas: What is the purpose of life? What is the goal of human existence? Certainly, we don't want to live to be 120 just to play golf or bingo for another half century. Ideally, we will find a way to extend our lives so additional years produce additional richness, so the quality of life continues to increase with time, so an increase in years means an increase in meaning, in understanding, in wisdom.

For this reason, an attempt to extend life arbitrarily and mechanically—with hormone shots, for example, or gene transplants—might be problematic. Even if we master them, such approaches might give us time without insight. We would live more years, but be no wiser. The current state of our society, produced by the current levels of wisdom available, certainly doesn't encourage us to feel that such mechanistic life extension would be an unalloyed blessing.

Right now the family basis of our society is unraveling, our streets are filled with crime, and our water and air are choked with pollution. Our economic system is faltering, our educational system is widely condemned, and our health care system is helping to bankrupt the nation while producing health and sickness in a disheartening ratio. These are the fruits of the current levels of intelligence and maturity available in our society. It's hard to believe we simply want more of the same.

It is also true that lengthening life span has already produced a generational crisis in modern societies. As the baby boom generation ages toward retirement, leaving behind a much smaller generational cohort to do the work and pay the bills, age-related friction is increasing in the society. Many younger people now feel that senior citizens are a drag on the nation, an unproductive segment of society with increasingly exorbitant health care bills. The value of the eldest generation has become lost in a cloud of financial concerns.

I believe that the consciousness-based health care provided by Maharishi Ayur-Ved can help enlighten society and resolve this generational tug-of-war. The same basic techniques of Maharishi Ayur-Ved which enhance physical health also raise the level of consciousness. With prevention-oriented natural approaches that nourish both body *and* mind, every year devoted to lengthening life is also spent growing rapidly toward enlightenment. The Vedic tradition has always maintained that this continued evolution will render the eldest generation the most judicious and discerning. Not only will the burden of their health care costs be dramatically reduced. Those most advanced in years will also be most advanced in the quality of consciousness. The oldest generation will also be the most valuable. With a leadership group that has spent long years developing the quality of their consciousness, we can look forward to a time when the problems of our society will be resolved much more effectively.

RESOLVING THE HEALTH CARE CRISIS

The most immediate social benefit of implementing Maharishi Ayur-Ved, however, will doubtless be a reduction of the crushing costs of health care. With costs spiraling out of control, governments are already taking drastic action. Most have adopted, or will soon adopt, variations of price control as a means to keep costs down. But no economist expects price controls to work as a long-term solution. Whenever prices are controlled, economic systems become distorted. Moreover, the history of price controls leads us to expect that as soon as they are released, rapid inflation takes place.

From an economic perspective, in fact, there is no real hope to contain costs in the long run while demand for health services continues to be high. In any undistorted market, supply and demand set the prices. If demand remains high, and the supply is relatively stable, prices remain high. This inexorable law underlies a nightmare scenario for the United States government. It wishes to extend medical coverage to the 37 million Americans not currently covered, but it fears increasing health care costs that will turn that coverage into an intolerable economic burden—and make a mockery of all efforts at deficit reduction. Unless something can be done to reduce health care demand, such a result seems inevitable.

Reducing demand has not been seriously considered, however, and for a simple reason: No one has known how to do it. People have continued to fall sick, and no wellness program has emerged that clearly keeps people healthy, that clearly cuts health care costs per person, or that even contains the rise of costs to any significant degree.

But that has changed now. The free radical paradigm—and the effective control of free radicals through Maharishi Ayur-Ved—have provided a thoroughly demonstrated approach for systematically cutting the demand for health care. In Chapter Six we saw the research demonstrating that the Transcendental Meditation technique by itself reduces health care costs by more than 10% each year (long-term meditators show a cumulative 50% reduction in health care utilization). We also reviewed the seven-year insurance study showing that people who control free radicals through an integrated approach—using Transcendental Meditation, Maharishi Amrit Kalash, and other aspects of Maharishi Ayur-Ved—go to the hospital for illness or surgery 80% less than the general population.

This research indicates that we have a potent technology for reducing the demand for health care services. By keeping people healthy through the control of free radicals, we can reduce the pressure on our health care system—and reduce health care costs in two ways. First, of course, individuals will require less care and run up lower costs. Second, the providers in the health care system, faced with fewer customers, will find themselves in competition for those who remain. In every market, such increased competition puts downward pressure on prices. If you can't sell your goods, you run a sale. The inexorable upward spiral of health care prices can be reversed.

A TIME FOR ACTION

It is true that rapid implementation of this program will require vision and courage from society's leaders. Attitudes and habits are difficult to change. Even many of us born in India, for example, have had to deal with a bias against an ancient, traditional health care system. I am sure the challenge is even greater for people to whom this system comes from halfway around the world. I also have personal experience of the scientist's biases in favor of isolated active ingredients and against complex herbal formulations, in favor of physical techniques based on a materialist paradigm and against mental techniques based on a consciousness paradigm. And I'm sure that nearly all of us have such an ingrained understanding of the pace of aging and illness that we can scarcely believe scientific research that shows—from simple techniques already tested—a better than 80% decline in serious illness.

But we live in an age of science. We need no longer give in to bias or preconception or failure of imagination. The research evidence indicates that, as individuals, we can take control of free radicals and take charge of our health. As societies, we can contain the damage of molecular attack and defuse the health care crisis.

More research should go forward, of course. But given the brutal damage caused by free radicals in every cell at every moment, there is no reason to sit idly by until the last experiment is completed. A well-documented anti-oxidant program is already available. It is hard to argue that we should continue to age and fall ill at our previous pace when we already know how to slow that pace dramatically.

I can only speak for myself. My investigations have brought me face to face again with the ayurvedic approach to health care long preserved in my homeland. I have obtained research results more dramatic than any I ever dared to dream. These results have led me to study the theoretical underpinnings of ayurveda—especially as they have been clarified by Maharishi Mahesh Yogi in Maharishi Ayur-Ved. My conclusion is that ayurveda provides to the current modalities of modern medicine a significant new program of prevention-oriented care.

The theory of ayurveda is more fundamental than any I know in medical science. It is based on a consciousness paradigm—an understanding only now being glimpsed by leading physicists and mathematicians. This theory provides an understanding for powerful preventive technologies that seem otherwise incomprehensibly effective.

In addition, the approaches of ayurveda are based on direct insights cognized within the profound awarenesses of sages who spent a lifetime using systematic technologies to refine the quality of their consciousness. Their discoveries, integrated and comprehensive, have now been validated through objective investigation. These results have redefined the possibilities of human life and health.

I, for one, believe that the evidence to date gives us a clear choice. Each of us can use simple techniques to transform both our physical and psychological health. Every society can adopt simple programs to resolve the health care crisis while also releasing creative energies that can recreate the nation.

We have completely new knowledge about human potential. Both the quality of our health and the extent of our fulfillment—as individuals and as nations—seem now just a matter of choice.

Resources

This book presents up-to-date and significant medical developments and research. No one, however, should read this book and attempt to treat a physical condition simply on that basis. If you are ill, consult a physician. For more information:

IN THE UNITED STATES

Doctors trained in Maharishi Ayur-Ved: For those who would like to consult a medical doctor who has also been trained in the approaches of Maharishi Ayur-Ved, a nationwide 800 number has been established.

Call: 1-800-THE-VEDA
             (in Massachusetts, the number is 1-508-368-1818)

Herbal supplements: Maharishi Ayur-Ved herbal food supplements are available as nutritional dietary supplements formulated under Ayur-Vedic protocol. They are offered by the formulators as a dietary supplement and for no other use or purpose.

Call: 1-800-ALL-VEDA
             (in Massachusetts the number is 1-508-368-1818)

Or write: Maharishi Ayur-Veda Products International
             P.O. Box 541
             Lancaster, MA 01523
             USA

Training programs: If you would like information on training programs in Maharishi Ayur-Ved,

Call: 1-515-472-1166

Or write: College of Maharishi Ayur-Ved at
             Maharishi International University
             Office of Admissions
             1000 North Fourth Street, DB 1155
             Fairfield, IA 52557-1155
             USA

IN CANADA

For information on Maharishi Ayur-Ved,

Call: 1-800-461-9685

Or write: Maharishi Ayur-Ved Information Service
            P.O. Box 6600
            Huntsville, Ontario POA 1KO
            Canada

IN THE UNITED KINGDOM

Call: 0800 269303, or
            0695 51015

Or write: Maharishi Ayur-Ved Products
            Peel House, Peel Road
            West Pimbo
            Skelmersdale
            Lancashire, WN8 9PT
            England

IN EUROPE

Call: 31 4752 3619
Fax: 31 4752 4055

Or write: Maharishi Ayur-Ved Products
            Groote Straat 27
            Vlodrop, The Netherlands 6063

IN AUSTRALIA

Call: 2-977 5066

Or write: Maharishi Ayur-Ved Health Centre
            68 Wood St., Manly
            Sydney, N.S.W., 2095

IN NEW ZEALAND

Call: 09 524 5883

Or write: MAP New Zealand
            9 Adam St, Greenlane
            Auckland

Index

Carbon monoxide, 61, 63
Carbon tetrachloride, 61-62, 117, 125
Cardiovascular disease,
    caused by free radicals, 82-87
    and Maharishi Amrit Kalash, 156-157
Cartilage
    and free radical damage, 91-92
Catalase, 32, 114-115
Cataracts, 24, 74
    and free radical damage, 94
Catechin, 129
Catecholamines, 66, 156, 270, 273, 317
Cathcart, Robert, 123
Cell differentiation and dysdif-
    ferentiation (see Differentiation
    and Dysdifferentiation)
Cell membrane, 43, 45-46, 118, 124, 143, 151, 152, 156
    and free radical damage, 79-81
    function of, 78-79
    structure of, 78
Cell receptors (see Receptors)
Cerebral blood flow
    during Transcendental Meditation, 179
Ceruloplasmin, 118-119, 123, 131
Charak Samhita, 207, 236
Chemical toxicity,
    and free radicals, 26-27, 60- 63, 68
    and Maharishi Amrit Kalash, 158-159
Chemotaxis, 55-59, 79, 83, 116-117, 129, 146, 151
Chemotherapy, 269
Chhandas, 241-243, 250-252, 258, 262-263, 265, 273, 292
Chlorpromazine, 61
Cholesterol, 1, 82-83, 147, 157, 188, 277, 287, 295-296
Chronobiology, 299
Clinical presentation, 73-74

Codon,
    in DNA, 76-77, 250, 252
Cognition, 214, 216, 226-227, 229-230, 292, 304, 307, 329
    definition of, 207-209, 230
    as basis of ayurveda, 207-209
Colitis, 74, 92
Collagen, 24, 61, 156-157
    and cancer growth, 91
    and rheumatoid arthritis, 91-92
Collagenases, 91
Consciousness, *passim*
    as basic approach of Maharishi
    Ayur-Ved, 278-282
    as basis of physical body, 257
    as basis of physical universe, 207-209, 218-224
    and physical health, 257-262
    as Samhita of Rishi, Devata, and
    Chhandas, 241
    self-interacting dynamics of, 240-242
    self-interacting dynamics give rise
    to manifest universe, 242-243
Consciousness paradigm, 11, 206, 231, 312, 328-329
    definition of, 3-4, 208-209
    and free radical paradigm, 236-238
    in terms of physics, 218-224
Constitution of the Universe, 248-249, 252
    in DNA, 249-252
    how the human mind can contact, 252-253
Cortisol, 66, 173, 190, 273
Creativity, 200, 221, 244, 323
Crohn's disease, 24, 74, 92
Crooke, Elliott, 20
Cytochrome oxidase, 51
Cytochrome P-450, 62
Cytoplasm, 289
Cytosine, 76
Cytoskeleton, 42, 74, 289
Cytosol, 42, 121